Topics in
Paediatric
Gastroenterology

Topics in Paediatric Gastroenterology

Edited by

Dr J A Dodge

Pitman Medical

First published 1976

PITMAN MEDICAL PUBLISHING CO LTD
42 Camden Road, Tunbridge Wells,
Kent TN1 2QD

Associated Companies

UNITED KINGDOM
Pitman Publishing Ltd, London
Focal Press Ltd, London

USA
Pitman Publishing Corporation, California
Fearon Publishers Inc, California

AUSTRALIA
Pitman Publishing Pty Ltd, Melbourne

CANADA
Pitman Publishing, Toronto
Copp Clark Publishing, Toronto

EAST AFRICA
Sir Isaac Pitman and Sons Ltd, Nairobi

SOUTH AFRICA
Pitman Publishing Co SA (Pty) Ltd, Johannesburg

NEW ZEALAND
Pitman Publishing NZ Ltd, Wellington

ISBN: 0 272 79375 2

Cat. No. 21 0657 81

Text set in 10/12 pt IBM Press Roman,
printed by photolithography,
and bound in Great Britain at The Pitman Press, Bath

Contents

Speakers

Dr J Apley
CBE, MD, FRCP — Consultant Paediatrician, United Bristol Hospitals

Dr J A Dodge
MD, FRCPE, DCH — Senior Lecturer, Department of Child Health, Welsh National School of Medicine, University Hospital of Wales, Cardiff

Professor H B Hadorn
MD (Zurich)
PhD (Melbourne) — Head of Gastrointestinal Unit, University Children's Hospital, Berne, Switzerland

Dr J Harries
MB, MRCP, DCH — Senior Lecturer in Paediatrics, Institute of Child Health, Guilford Street, London

Dr K W Heaton,
MD, FRCP — Consultant Senior Lecturer in Medicine, University of Bristol

Mr E R Howard
MS, FRCS — Consultant Surgeon, King's College Hospital, London S E 5

Mr J Lari
MB, FRCS — Consultant Paediatric Surgeon, University Hospital of Wales, Cardiff

Dr B W Lawrie
MB, DMRD, FFR — Department of Diagnostic Radiology, University Hospital of Wales, Cardiff

Dr A S McNeish
MB, MRCP — Senior Lecturer in Child Health, University of Birmingham

Dr J Morris
MB, MRCP — Consultant Physician, Bridgend General Hospital

Dr A Mowat
MB, MRCP,
DObstRCOG, DCH — Consultant Paediatrician, King's College Hospital, London S E 5

Dr P Pinkerton
MD, FRCP, DPM — Senior Consultant and Lecturer in Paediatric Psychiatry, University of Liverpool

Dr J Polak
MD, MRCPath — Lecturer in Histochemistry, Royal Postgraduate Medical School, Hammersmith Hospital, London

Dr Henry Ryley
PhD — Senior Scientific Officer, Dept. of Medical Microbiology, Welsh National School of Medicine, University Hospital of Wales, Cardiff

Dr M Shiner
FRCP, DCH — Consultant Gastroenterologist, M R C Gastroenterology Unit, Central Middlesex Hospital, London

Dr J R Sibert
MA, MB, MRCP,
DObstRCOG — Senior Registrar, Department of Paediatrics, Llandough Hospital, Cardiff

Dr E Thompson
MD, FRCP, DCH — Senior Lecturer, Department of Child Health, Welsh National School of Medicine

Participants

Dr A Alwyn-Smith	Orchard Cottage, Newton, Porthcawl, Glam.
Dr L J H Arthur	Consultant Paediatrician, Derbyshire Children's Hospital
Dr J W T Benson	Paediatric Registrar, Royal Berkshire Hospital, Reading
Dr M Blair	Senior Registrar in Medical Paediatrics, Royal Hospital for Sick Children, Glasgow
Dr G Brown	Bryn Gwyn, Mount Pleasant, Fleur-de-Lys, Blackwood, Gwent
Dr D Burman	Consultant Paediatrician, Bristol Royal Hospital for Sick Children, St Michael's Hill, Bristol
Dr C E Castillo	c/o The British Council, 10 Spring Gardens, London, SW1A 2BN
Dr P Crowle	Lecturer in Child Health, Southmead Hospital Bristol
Dr J M Davies	Consultant Paediatrician, Grimsby & Louth Hospital, Humberside
Professor E E Doyle	National Children's Hospital, Harcourt Street, Dublin 2
Dr J E Ellis	Paediatric Tutor, University of Manchester
Dr A R H El-Mufti	Research Fellow, Institute of Child Health, Francis Road, Birmingham 16
Dr Rosemary Evans	Paediatric Registrar, Southmead Hospital, Bristol
Dr T J Evans	Senior Registrar in Paediatrics, Cardiff Royal Infirmary
Dr J G Fleming	Senior Registrar in Paediatrics, Bristol Royal Hospital for Sick Children, St Michael's Hill, Bristol
Dr W R Forbes	Consultant Paediatrician, Glantawe Hospital, Swansea
Mr N V Freeman	Consultant Paediatric Surgeon, Southampton General Hospital
Dr J F T Glasgow	Senior Lecturer in Child Health, Queen's University, Belfast, N.I.
Dr A D Griffiths	Consultant Paediatrician, Nevill Hall Hospital, Abergavenny, Gwent
Dr A M Hood	182 Commercial Road, Newport, Gwent
Dr Frances Howard	Paediatric Registrar, St Peter's Hospital, Chertsey, Surrey

Dr C A Hughes	Paediatric Lecturer, Guy's Hospital, London
Dr Iyngkaran Nagalingam	Research Fellow, c/o East Birmingham Hospital, Bordesley Green East, Birmingham
Dr Penelope Johnson	75a High Street, Sutton Courtenay, Oxon.
Dr Keitel	U.S.A.A.F. Hospital Base, Frankfurt, W.Germany
Dr D M Lewis	Consultant Paediatrician, Bronglais Hospital, Aberystwyth, Dyfed.
Dr J M Littlewood	Consultant Paediatrician, Seacroft Hospital, York Road, Leeds
Dr D J Lloyd	Lecturer in Child Health, University of Aberdeen
Dr M P Mahoney	Consultant Physician, Blackburn Royal Infirmary, Blackburn
Dr S T Meller	Senior Registrar, Queen Mary's Hospital for Children, Carshalton, Surrey
Dr P McInerney	Clontarf, Caerleon Road, Llanfrechfa, Cwmbran, Gwent
Dr R B McGucken	Consultant Paediatrician, Royal Infirmary, Wigan
Dr H M I Nazer	R M O, Hospital for Sick Children, Tadworth, Surrey
Dr R Nelson	Consultant Paediatrician, Royal Victoria Infirmary, Newcastle upon Tyne
Dr A Palit	Consultant Paediatrician, Haverfordwest, Dyfed.
Dr R Prosser	Consultant Paediatrician, Royal Gwent Hospital, Newport, Gwent.
Dr G Roberts	Caerwent, Gwent.
Dr M B R Roberts	Senior Paediatric Registrar, Radcliffe Infirmary, Oxford
Dr Mary Rossiter	Consultant Paediatrician, North Middlesex Hospital, Silver Street, London, N 18
Dr N Rutter	Paediatric Registrar, Nottingham City Hospital
Dr Sonia San Martin	Clinical Research Fellow, Institute of Child Health, Francis Road, Birmingham
Dr E E Saelzer	Research Fellow in Paediatric Gastroenterology, Queen Elizabeth Hospital for Children, Hackney, London E 4.
Dr T M Scott	Paediatric Registrar, Royal Hospital for Sick Children, Yorkhill, Glasgow
Dr S K Sengupta	Paediatric S H O, County Hospital, Haverfordwest, Dyfed.
Dr B A M Smith	Consultant Paediatrician, Northern General Hospital, Sheffield

Dr O Troughton	Consultant Paediatrician, Pontefract General Infirmary, Pontefract
Dr C Upjohn	Consultant Paediatrician, Farnborough Hospital, Orpington, Kent
Dr J A Walker-Smith	Senior Lecturer and Consultant Paediatrician, Queen Elizabeth Hospital for Children, Hackney, London
Dr J L Wilkins	Consultant Paediatrician, St Mary's Hospital, Eastbourne, Sussex
Dr R G Wilson	Consultant Paediatrician, Kingston Hospital, Kingston-on-Thames, Surrey

Development of the Gut in the Fetus and Young Child

Development of Enzyme Systems in the Exocrine Pancreas and Small Intestine

B HADORN, M CWERN, B FRIOLET and R MARTIN DU PAN
Gastrointestinal Unit, Department of Paediatrics, University of Berne, Berne, Switzerland

For a better understanding of the disease processes which may alter the activity of intestinal and pancreatic enzymes, it is important to know the sequence of events in normal development. Although the various steps in development are guided by genetic mechanisms, environmental influences (e.g. hormonal or nutritional) may modify enzymatic activity during development.

PANCREATIC ENZYMES

Animal Experiments on Pancreatic Development

Rutter and his colleagues have investigated the development of the pancreas in mouse embryos and have proposed a model involving three regulatory events (Figure 1).

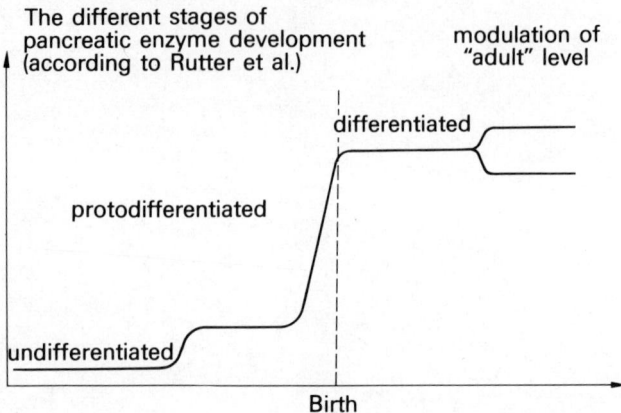

Figure 1

During early embryonic life the pancreas is in the undifferentiated state during which no specific enzyme synthesis takes place. With the appearance of the first zymogen granules in exocrine cells very low levels of pancreatic enzymes can be detected and these enzymes do not differ in their biochemical characteristics from the mature pancreatic enzymes. This state is called the proto-differentiated state. In most mammals and also in birds a dramatic increase of specific activity of these enzymes occurs shortly before birth and this is the result of a rapidly increased enzyme synthesis (the preformed enzymes are manufactured in greater amounts). After birth, the differentiated level is reached and enzymatic activity becomes more constant. However, nutritional and hormonal influences may still 'modulate' this level. This is not a developmental process but involves regulation of enzyme synthesis and turnover by extrinsic exogenous factors.

The human exocrine pancreas is morphologically well developed at birth, although the predominance of the endocrine tissue which is characteristic for the fetal pancreas is still visible. The functional capacity of the human newborn pancreas has been measured by Zoppi et al (1972) and it has been shown that the amounts of enzymes secreted are sufficient for hydrolysis of the food substances offered to the newborn child. One exception to this is pancreatic amylase which − according to many authors − is low at birth and develops slowly during the first year of life (see also Figure 2). Zoppi has also shown that the human pancreas shortly after birth is able to respond to hormonal and nutritional stimuli. Of great interest is Zoppi's finding that amylase activity was higher in newborns receiving starch rich food than in a control group of children who received an isocaloric amount of glucose during the same developmental period (Zoppi et al, 1973).

Very recently it has been suggested that in some newborn babies pancreatic exocrine function may be insufficient in relation to the amount of food offered to these babies (Robinson & Elliott, 1975) but this suggestion has been made on the basis of measurements of faecal trypsin and chymotrypsin which does not allow a precise estimation of pancreatic function.

In discussing disturbed exocrine pancreatic function of the newborn or the premature child, it is important to remember that the organ does not yet possess the enormous reserve capacity present in adult life. In children with congenital pancreatic insufficiency, symptoms such as failure to thrive, diarrhoea and hypoproteinaemia are frequent. Symptoms may become less pronounced later in life. The very high growth velocity of the newborn and the even greater growth velocity of prematures and small for dates necessitates intact exocrine pancreatic function.

Figure 3 shows a comparison between protein intakes of healthy children up to 24 months of age and also shows the rapidly decreasing growth velocity during this same period. It is possible that a deficiency of an intestinal or pancreatic enzyme which may limit the digestive capacity for protein manifests itself on a

3

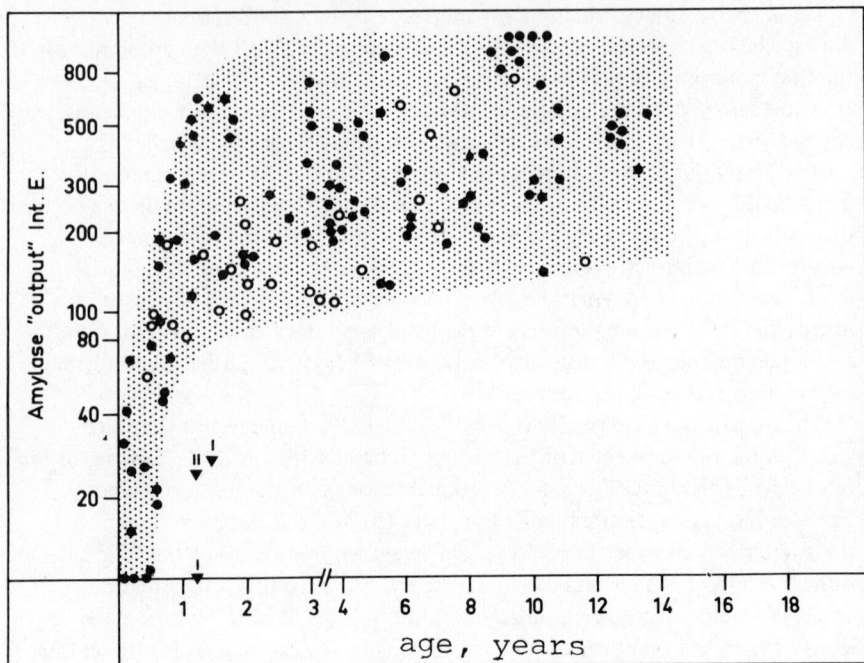

Figure 2. Pancreozymin-Secretin-Test: Amylase output in relation to age
- ● control patients (n = 109)
- ○ patients with malabsorption not due to pancreatic insufficiency (n = 28)
- ▼ 2 patients with clinical signs of starch intolerance and pancreatic amylase deficiency

In patient 1 three investigations were performed at the age of 4 months (not shown), 13 months and 17 months. Only after the age of 13 months was there an increase of amylase output but normal levels were never reached.

clinical level only during the first few months of life. Together with Haworth we have encountered this phenomenon in children with intestinal enterokinase deficiency (Haworth et al, 1975)

PANCREATIC AMYLASE DEFICIENCY

Dorothy Andersen (1942) and Shwachman et al (1943) have already stated that pancreatic amylase in the newborn is low and develops slowly during the first year of life. One of us has described amylase deficiency as a cause of chronic diarrhoea in infants (Martin Du Pan & Infante, 1961). In all patients the leading clinical symptom was fermentative diarrhoea and retardation of growth and weight increment while on a starch containing food. Similar observations have recently been made by Lillibridge and Townes (1973). We had the opportunity to investigate two patients with this disorder and in one patient it was possible to measure pancreatic function three times (Figure 1). The results of total

4

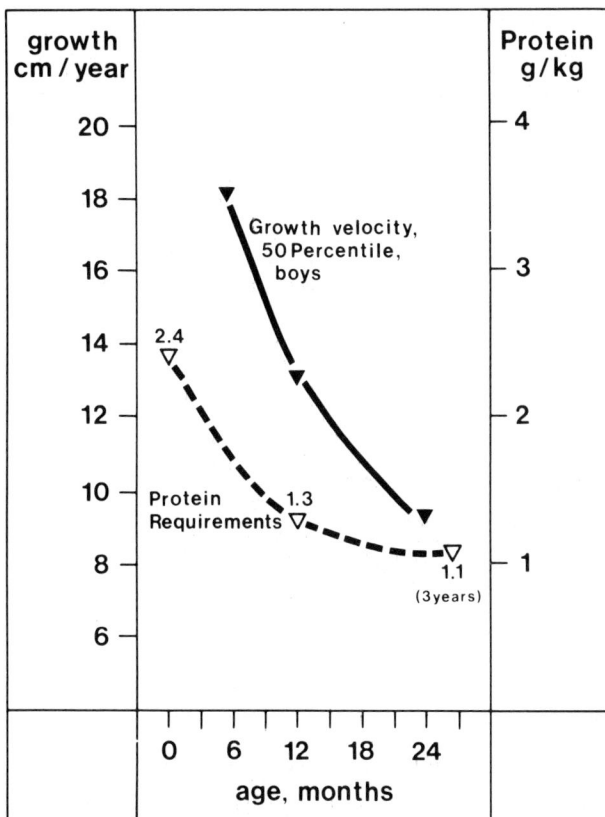

Figure 3. Growth velocity and protein requirement in infants between 0 and 26 months of age.

amylase output are shown in Figure 1, which also shows the development of amylase output in 137 children with and without malabsorption. Amylase deficiency may be a genetically determined disease as has been suggested by Martin Du Pan because several members of one family observed in Geneva have shown symptoms of starch intolerance (Figure 4).

Since pancreatic amylase occurs in different molecular forms, we have been interested to investigate the development of the various amylase isoenzymes in patients with amylase deficiency. A zymogram of pancreatic amylase is shown in Figure 5 in one of our patients with low amylase activity. Despite the differences in total activity, the isoenzyme pattern was the same during development of amylase activity in this patient. It appears thus that the total synthesis of amylase rather than the synthesis of single iso-enzymes is retarded in these children. It is important to differentiate pancreatic amylase deficiency from gluten induced enteropathy (coeliac disease). The criteria which permit this differentiation are listed in Table I.

5

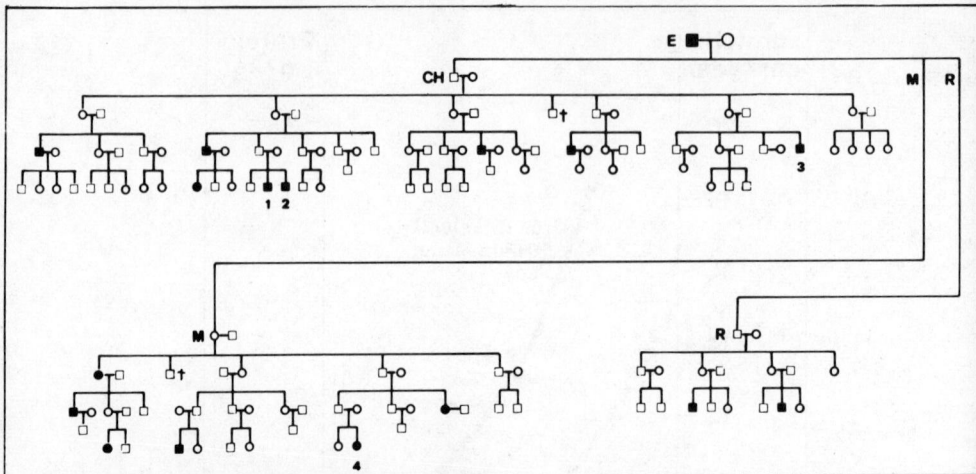

Figure 4. Pedigree of family M. from Geneva
■ subjects affected by starch intolerance
○
The pedigree suggests an autosomal dominant mode of inheritance.
1, 2, 3, 4 patients investigated with oral starch loads

TABLE I. Differential diagnosis
pancreatic
amylase   ↔   coeliac
deficiency   disease

	Pancreatic amylase deficiency	Coeliac disease
onset	immediately after first exposure to starch	some time after first exposure to gliadin
growth	usually normal	retarded
weight increment	slower while on starch containing diet	retarded
faeces	fermentative diarrhoea, low pH, Lugol positive, Clinitest positive	steatorrhoea, bulky stools, occasionally obstipation
small intestinal biopsy	normal morphology	abnormal morphology
pancreatic function test	isolated deficiency of amylase	normal
duration	transient, developmental problem	permanent

6

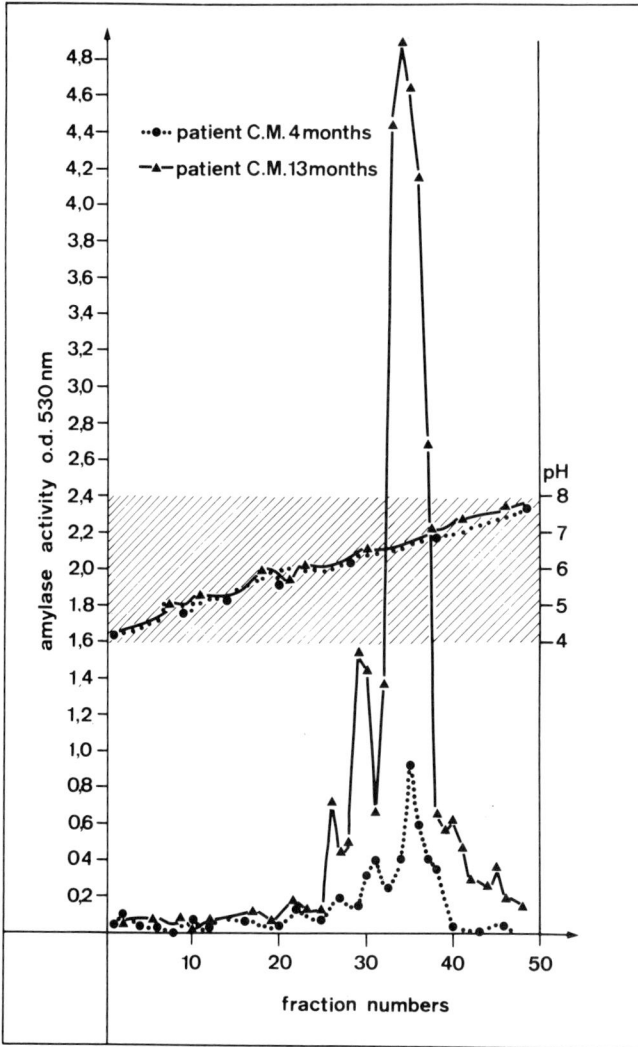

Figure 5. Isoenzymes of pancreatic α-amylase separated by isoelectric focusing in patient
C.M. at 4 months ---•--- and at 13 months —▲—
The isoelectric points of the isoenzymes vary between 5.5 and 8.

The therapy of amylase deficiency is straightforward. It is sufficient to replace dietary starch by disaccharides and the children will start to thrive immediately.

No cases of permanent amylase-deficiency have been known so far. In most patients amylase activity reaches normal levels between the age of two and three years.

Sucrase Activity

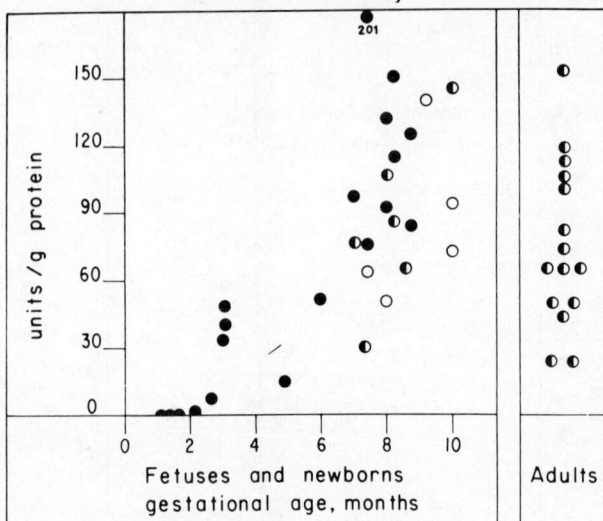

● = younger than 1 day

○ = older than 1 day, before first feeding

◑ = older than 1 day, after first feeding

Figure 6. Sucrase activity in human fetuses and newborns.

Lactase Activity

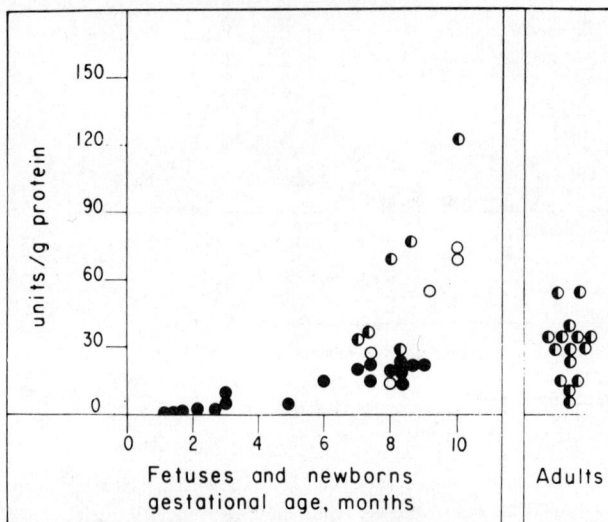

● = younger than 1 day

○ = older than 1 day, before first feeding

◑ = older than 1 day, after first feeding

Figure 7. Lactase activity in human fetuses and newborns.

8

INTESTINAL ENZYMES

The development of intestinal enzymes has been studied in great detail by many groups of workers. Auricchio and Rubino (1965) have studied the development of the disaccharidases. Lindberg et al (1975) have studied the development of dipeptidases and a great number of workers including Kretschmer (1972) and Koldovski (1969) have studied the development of lactase.

Sucrase-isomaltase activity as shown in Figure 6 increases between the third and the seventh month of gestation in man. At birth the activity (expressed in units per gram protein) is the same as in adults. Lactase-activity (Figure 7) shows essentially the same developmental curve, but in some newborns and in most prematures lactase-activity may be lower compared with the period shortly after birth. Lifshitz et al (1971) have suggested that this relatively low lactase-activity has clinical significance and may be responsible for the development of fermentative diarrhoea and metabolic acidosis if the diet of the child contains great amounts of lactose (human milk). Although this may be the case in some children these findings should not lead us to recommend complete replacement of lactose by glucose or other carbohydrates in the industrially made formulas for prematures and newborns. The slight fermentative diarrhoea of the breast fed child with its low stool pH and excretion of reducing substances (Davidson & Mullinger, 1970) is a physiological phenomenon and the rather acid environment in the colon of these babies may contribute to the development and maintenance of the physiological symbiont flora.

Lactase

a) *Congenital deficiency of intestinal lactase* is an extremely rare disorder and only a few cases have been documented after Holzel's and Durand's original descriptions (Holzel, Schwartz & Sutcliffe, 1959; Durand, 1958; Asp et al, 1973)

b) *selective adult type hypolactasia*   A different type of lactase deficiency is the specific hypolactasia of older children and adults which has been studied extensively by many authors in different ethnic groups throughout the world. Feeding of lactose in high doses to individuals with this type of lactase deficiency does not increase the enzymatic activity (Rosensweig, 1973). This is in contrast to sucrase-isomaltase malabsorption because a slight increase in enzymatic activity following feeding of sucrose and fructose was achieved in one patient by Rosenzweig.

The mechanisms by which low lactase activity in congenital lactase deficiency is achieved has been discussed by Asp and colleagues (1973). Interestingly, the residual enzymatic activity in the subjects with congenital lactase deficiency was lower than that in older children and adults with selective hypolactasia deficiency. This has prompted these authors to suggest a different mechanism to be responsible for the low lactase activity in these two groups of patients.

9

We recently analysed the composition of the brush border membrane in two patients with the adult type lactase deficiency and in two cases of congenital lactase deficiency and no difference in the composition of the brush border membrane glycoproteins was detected, e.g. the peak corresponding to lactase activity was reduced in both instances (Freiburghaus et al, 1976). The reduction of the amount of protein corresponded approximately to the reduction of specific activity of lactase. Similar findings have been reported from Crane's group (Crane et al, 1975).

Congenital lactase deficiency may become a severe clinical problem if the lactose content of the milk is high, but how about the adult type lactase deficiency? How important is it clinically? Occasionally we have observed patients who develop severe borborygmi and very loose stools with flatulence following ingestion of as little as one glass of milk. A particularly striking example has recently been published (Ahmed, 1975). In these subjects the use of a lactose-free milk (AL 110 Nestlé) or the complete elimination of lactose from the diet is indicated. We suspect that the clinical importance of the low lactase activity in some ethnic groups has been exaggerated mainly by the paramedical press. Some of these subjects are able to tolerate low amounts of lactose. A milk with a reduced lactose content is probably indicated in children who suffer in addition to their genetically low lactase activity from gastrointestinal infections and further reduction of the enzymatic activity. This problem is being investigated but it should not be advocated a priori to use a lactose-free milk for the total population of children with kwashiorkor before the clinical importance of the low lactase activity has been clearly established in this population of children. In no instance should the distribution of milk powder to children with kwashiorkor be delayed because of a 'lactase' problem. A more important problem is protein deficiency and dry milk powder is an excellent source of this important nutrient which can be used whenever the possibility of reconstitution of the milk in a hygienic environment is given.

Sucrase-isomaltase Malabsorption

This disorder occurs with a greater frequency than congenital lactase deficiency and follows an autosomal recessive mode of inheritance (Kerry & Townley, 1965). Recently it has been suggested by Dubs, Steinmann and Gitzelmann (1973) that patients with sucrase-isomaltase deficiency may be able to synthesise a precursor of sucrase (catalytically inactive antigen CIA) which is detectible with immunological methods.

Dubs (1974) has also documented in rabbits that CIA develops earlier in embryonic life than the active sucrase-isomaltase complex (Figure 8). It is possible therefore to postulate that sucrose-isomaltose malabsorption represents an example of a developmental problem in which the conversion of the catalytically inactive precursor of sucrase to the fully active molecule is not possible. In one

10

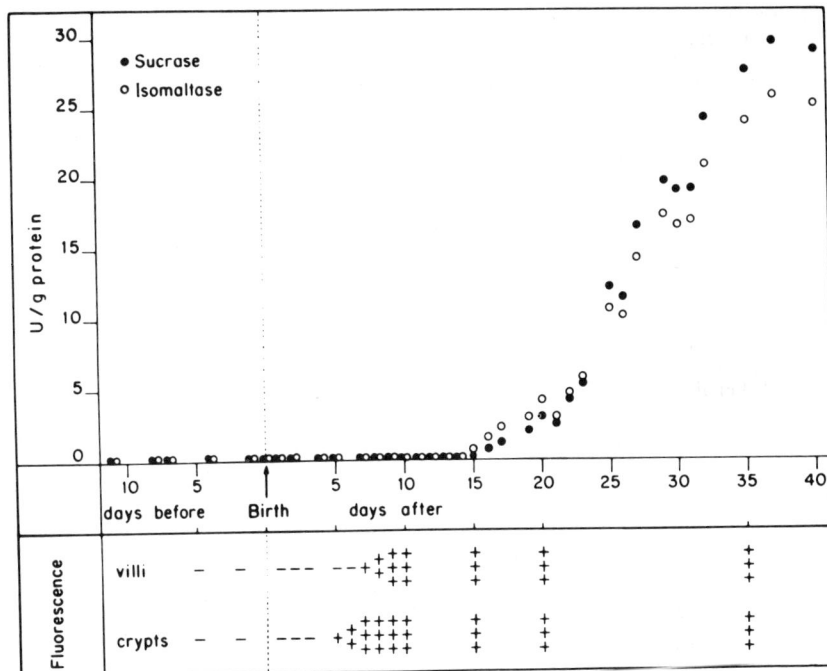

Figure 8. Development of intestinal sucrase and isomaltase activity in the guinea pig.
According to Dubs. The catalytically inactive antigen (CIA) as detected by
specific immunofluorescence appears earlier than the enzymatic activity.

such patient with immunologically demonstrable CIA we have recently found
that there is complete deletion of the glycoprotein corresponding to the sucrase-
isomaltase activity on polyacrylamid gels made from semi-purified brush border
membrane fragments. The polyacrylamid gels showed the appearance of a band
which was not seen in control patients without sucrase-isomaltase deficiency.
This additional band may represent an altered sucrase-isomaltase complex or
possibly one of the two subunits of this enzyme. Preiser et al (1974) and Schmitz
et al (1974) have also demonstrated the absence of the characteristic sucrase-
isomaltase band from polyacrylamid gels but no additional band was found in
these patients. It is possible therefore that different types of this disorder may
exist with different molecular mechanisms leading to the defective enzymatic
activity. It is certain that the new techniques of analysis of the glycoproteins of
the brush border membrane which have been introduced by Schmitz, and
Maestracchi et al (1975) working in Crane's laboratory will lead to a better understanding of the molecular mechanisms involved in the production of congenital
intestinal enzyme deficiencies.

11

References

Ahmed, H F (1975), *Lancet, ii*, 319.
Andersen, D H (1942) *American Journal of Diseases of Children, 63*, 643.
Asp, N-G et al (1973) *Lancet, ii*, 329.
Auricchio, S et al (1965) *Pediatrics, 35*, 944.
Cock, G C (1973) In *Symposia of The Swedish Nutrition Foundation XI*. (Ed.) B Borgström,
  A Dahlqvist and L Hambraeus. Almqvist & Wiksell, Uppsala, Page 52.
Crane, R K et al (1976) In *Membranes and Diseases*. (Ed). Bolis, Hoffman & Leaf, International
  Conference on Biological Membranes (to be published)
Davidson, A G F and Mullinger, M (1970) *Pediatrics, 46*, 632.
Dubs, R (1974) Ph D Thesis, University of Zurich.
Dubs, R et al (1973) *Helvetica Paediatrica Acta, 28*, 187.
Durand, P (1958) *Minerva Pediatrica, 10*, 706.
Freiburghaus, A et al (1976) *New England Journal of Medicine*, (In press)
Haworth, J C et al (1975) *Archives of Disease in Childhood, 50*, 277.
Holzel, A et al (1959) *Lancet, i*, 1126.
Kerry, K R and Townley, R R W (1965) *Australian Paediatric Journal, 1*, 223.
Koldovsky, O (1969) *Development of the Functions of the Small Intestine in Mammals and
  Man*. S. Karger, Basel.
Kretchmer, N (1972) *Scientific American, 4*, 70
Lifshitz, F et al (1971) *Pediatric Research, 5*, 213
Lillibridge, C B and Townes, P L (1973) *Journal of Pediatrics, 82*, 279
Lindberg, T et al (1975) In *Peptide Transport in Protein Nutrition*. (Ed) D M Matthews and
  J W Payne. North Holland Publishing Company, Amsterdam. Page 204.
Maestracci, D et al (1975) *Biochimica et Biophysica Acta, 382*, 147
Martin Du Pan, R and Infante, F (1961) *Internationale Zeitschrift fur Vitaminforschrung,
  1*, 67
Preiser, H et al (1974) *Biochimica et Biophysica Acta, 363*, 279
Robinson, P G and Elliott, R B (1975) *Lancet, ii*, 817
Rosensweig, N S (1973) In *Symposia of The Swedish Nutrition Foundation XI*. (Ed)
  B Borgström, A Dahlqvist and L Hambraeus. Almqvist & Wiksell, Uppsala. Page 21.
Rutter, W J et al (1967) *Experimental Biology and Medicine, 1*, 118. S Karger, Basel.
Schmitz, J et al (1974) *Biomedicine, 21*, 440
Schmitz, J et al (1975) In *Pädiatrische Fortbildungskurse für die Praxis*. Vol.42. S Karger,
  Basel. Page 13
Schwachman, H et al (1943) *American Journal of Diseases of Children, 66*, 418
Zoppi, G et al (1972) *Pediatric Research, 6*, 880
Zoppi, G et al (1973) *Pediatric Research, 7*, 198

Discussion

PROFESSOR E D WILLIAMS Is there evidence as to whether CIA is a sucragen
or a prosucrase?

HADORN It is not a prosucrase in the sense that it is a proenzyme which by
proteolytic action is converted into an active enzyme. We believe that there
are two moieties, one is the sucrase moiety S, and one is the isomaltase moiety
I. Both of them have a molecular weight of approximately 1100. Each of them
carries an active centre somewhere. One can ac...ally separate the two moieties
of the sucrase-isomaltase complex, in alkaline conditions, and then investigate
them separately. Now what happens during embryonic life is not absolutely
certain but one thing which is possible is that chains are synthesised separately

12

and are then put together. One could explain in this way why there was no band in the area of 22,000 molecular weight, because the chain separates. It could be that in sucrase-isomaltase insufficiency, the two moieties have been synthesised, but they have not been put together properly. Now comes the question, why is the antibody able to detect a sucrase molecule before it becomes active? A very simple explanation can be that the active centre has nothing to do with the antibody combining side. We may imagine that the antibody combines with the antibody combining site and that the antibody combining site is not affected by the mutation. The mutation would always affect the active centre. Dahlquist also finds CIA in sucrase-isomaltase enzyme insufficiency.

WILLIAMS Is there any morphological change — does it accumulte in any way? There is some evidence that the precursor of alpha-1-antitrypsin accumulates in the liver in deficiency states. Does *this* accumulate in the gut?

HADORN There is no evidence. All one can say is that in immunofluorescent studies in a normal child, you have immunofluorescence all along the brush-border. In the sucrase-isomaltase deficient child, you also have this immuno-fluoresence but it is a little bit more diffuse.

13

Meconium: Its Origins, Composition and Abnormalities

H C RYLEY

Meconium is the term given to the first stools passed after birth and represents the accumulation of the intestinal contents during fetal life. A meconium-like plug of material may be seen in the colon as early as the fourth month of fetal life (Windle, 1971) but such early accumulations represent only a small proportion of the final meconial mass. Meconium is characteristically dark in colour, mucilaginous, sterile and odourless. It disappears by the fourth day after birth.

This paper describes the origin of meconium components and their distribution both in health and disease. Aspects of meconium composition have previously been reviewed by Smith (1959) and Schultze and Heremans (1966).

ORIGIN OF MECONIUM

The components of meconium originate from many sources. Apart from the active secretions of the alimentary tract mucosa that contribute the bulk of the final meconial mass, there is a passive transudate from the vascular system of the gut and secretions from the bile and pancreatic ducts. Amniotic fluid provides another source of material, for a fetus ingests amniotic fluid equivalent to 10% of its own body weight per day as early as at four months of fetal life (Pritchard, 1966). This represents less than 10 ml at four months but the volume of amniotic fluid ingested per day is more than 500 ml at term. Amniotic fluid not only contains material synthesised in situ by the amnion but also contains constituents from fetal bronchial secretions and urine, together with a substantial maternal vascular transudate (Schultze & Heremans, 1966). The composition of meconium does not accurately reflect a mixture of these secretions and fluids because meconium composition is affected by water reabsorption and intrinsic enzymatic activity during its agglomeration in the colon. Also, it has been shown that during the fourth to seventh month of intrauterine life, part of the gut content is accumulated within the epithelial cells forming ovoid bodies; these 'meconium corpuscles' are eliminated later back into the gut lumen after their exposure to cellular lysosomal activity (Andersen et al, 1964; Schwidt, 1971). Whether the above has any marked effect on the final composition of meconium is as yet unclear.

14

COMPOSITION OF MECONIUM

Meconium has a water content of about 70–75% of the total wet weight (Hall & O'Toole, 1934). Seventy to eighty percent of the solid phase is composed of mucin and related glycopeptides with both plasma proteins and tissue debris contributing a further 5–10% of the total dry weight. The rest of the dry weight is made up of enzymes and small molecular weight components such as ions, haemoglobin metabolites, steroids and sterols. The composition of meconium will be considered in more detail below, and unless otherwise stated the details concern meconium collected from healthy neonates.

Tissue Debris

Most of the tissue debris is composed of desquamations of the fetal alimentary tract, mouth and skin as well as vernix debris and lanugo hair (Smith, 1959). It was identification of these latter two components in meconium in the late nineteenth century which first established that the human fetus ingested amniotic fluid although such evidence was not generally accepted until the advent of x-ray techniques (Becker et al, 1940).

Enzymes

Table I illustrates many of the enzymes identified in meconium and they may be classified into two main groups, proteolytic and glycosidic enzymes.

The basic proteolytic enzymes such as trypsin and chymotrypsin which originate from the pancreas have an important role in the formation of the final composition of meconium. Not only do they degrade most of the soluble proteins present initially in the gut contents but they act also on the mucins secreted by the mucosa, liberating water soluble fragments and consequently reducing the viscosity of the mucilaginous phase. The absence of proteolytic enzymes may in part be responsible for meconium ileus: ileal obstruction by impacted viscid meconium. Although basic proteolytic activity can be demonstrated in all meconium specimens from healthy infants, some workers have been unable to detect either specific tryptic or chymotryptic activity in all specimens (Eggermont, 1966) while other workers have not reported this difficulty (Schachter & Dixon, 1965). Slight acidic protease activity may be also detected (Schwarz, 1953; Ryley, unpublished), although the origin of these enzymes, whether gastric or lysosomal, is uncertain.

The other main group of enzymes, the glycosidases, mainly originate from the intestinal mucosa (Eggermont, 1966). Eggermont has shown that as glycosidases are liable to proteolysis, their final concentration in meconium is dependent on the degree of intrinsic proteolytic activity present.

15

TABLE I. Enzymes in Meconium

I. *Proteolytic Enzymes*

Trypsin	Schachter and Dixon (1965) Eggermont (1966)
Chymotrypsin	Schachter and Dixon (1965) Eggermont (1966)
Rennin	Schwarz (1953)
Dipeptidases	Schwarz (1953)
Acidic Proteases	Schwarz (1953) Ryley (unpublished)

II. *Glycosidase*

Maltase	Eggermont (1966)
Isomaltase	Eggermont (1966)
Sucrase	Eggermont (1966)
Lactase	Eggermont (1966)
Trehalase	Eggermont (1966)

III. *Lysosomal Enzymes*

Alkaline Phosphatase	Eggermont (1966)

Mucins and Glycopeptides

Although the mucins and related glycopeptides constitute the bulk of the dry meconial mass, remarkably little work has been carried out to characterise these substances. In the early fifties, Buchanan and Rapoport (1951) isolated fractions with blood group activity and with compositions similar to other epithelial mucins. No further work was reported until 1964 when Kimura and Nagai described the isolation of three water soluble sialoglycopeptide fractions; all fractions had blood group activity. More recently, Fraser and Clamp (1975) reported the separation of two glycoprotein fractions together with an insoluble fraction left after water extraction. One water soluble glycoprotein fraction had blood group activity although glycoprotein fractions containing H activity had a significantly lower molecular weight than those containing A or B activity. The other glycoprotein fraction was characterised by containing mannose, a sugar usually absent in epithelial mucins.

I have also been studying the composition of the mucin ground substance of meconium and have to date characterised five distinct fractions using antiserum to meconium and various fractionation procedures. The antiserum had been absorbed with human serum protein and gave no precipitation lines against human serum. One fraction was *water-insoluble* and resistant to proteolysis by trypsin; it represents 30–40% of the whole mucilaginous phase and is similar to that described by Fraser and Clamp. The *water soluble* glycopeptides may be separated

16

into two groups according to their solubility in ammonium sulphate. Three components could be demonstrated in the ammonium sulphate-insoluble fraction; two gave strong precipitation arcs with immunoelectrophoresis against anti-meconium serum. A third component gave only a faint arc against the antiserum but may be separated from the other two fractions on a column of Sepharose 4B. The ammonium sulphate-soluble fraction constituted about half of the total water-soluble glycopeptides and gave no detectable precipitation arc against anti-meconium serum. It could, however, be separated into sulphate, sialic acid and fucose rich fractions similar to those previously described for bronchial secretions (Ryley, 1972). This suggests that at least some of the meconium mucins are similar to other epithelial mucins and contain a mixture of sulpho-, sialo-, and fucomucins, prior to intrinsic proteolysis.

Serum Proteins

The absolute identification of serum proteins in meconium from healthy neonates was first described by Roulet and von Muralt (1961) who reported that immuno-electrophoretic analysis of meconium against human serum anti-serum gave 4–5 arcs, two identified as due to albumin and γ-globulin and two further unidentified α-arcs. Schachter and Dixon (1965) reported that they were unable to detect serum proteins in many of their meconium specimens from healthy infants. More recently Ryley, et al (1974) reported the identification of two precipitation arcs due to α_1-antitrypsin and α_1-antichymotrypsin in all specimens analysed (Figure 1); from the analysis of one hundred specimens, the content of α_1-antitrypsin and α_1-antichymotrypsin was 48.4 ± 23.8 mg and 4.0 ± 2.7 mg per gram dry weight respectively (Ryley et al, 1975). About 5% of specimens contained more than 1 mg of albumin per gram dry weight and transferrin, Gc globulin, α_2-HS and IgG were found in less than 0.5% of specimens. There is a difference of opinion as to the major source of serum proteins in meconium. I would suggest that the major source of serum proteins in meconium is from ingested amniotic fluid with a small contribution from the passive transudates from the underlying vascular system of the gut; other workers hold that the passive transudate is the most important source (Kaiser, Shwachman; personal communications). Normally most of the serum protein, whatever its source, is destroyed by intrinsic proteolysis with the exception of the protease inhibitors. Numerous serum proteins can be found in meconium up to 22 weeks of fetal life (Ryley, unpublished).

One glycoprotein of non-serum origin has recently been isolated from meconium; Rule and Goleski-Reilly (1973) isolated carcinoembryonic antigen (CEA) from meconium of healthy infants born at full term. It is present in meconium at a concentration of about 0.1 mg per gram of protein and has some antigen differences from CEA isolated from tumour tissue.

17

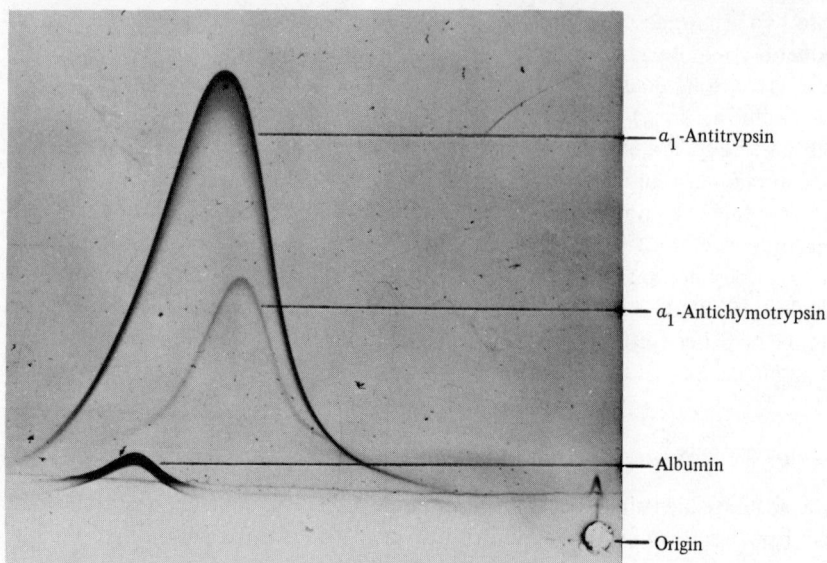

Figure 1. Crossed immunoelectrophoretic pattern of meconium from a healthy neonate against rabbit antihuman serum. Electrophoresis and staining were carried out by methods previously described (Ryley et al, 1974). Apart from arcs due to α_1-antitrypsin and α_1-antichymotrypsin which are found in all specimens from healthy infants, a small arc due to albumin may also be seen. Such an albumin arc is found in about 5% of specimens from healthy neonates.

Small Molecular Components

Ions

Widdowson, et al (1962) described the estimation of calcium, magnesium, and strontium and found that the magnesium and calcium concentrations were similar. By comparing strontium and calcium ion concentrations in amniotic fluid and meconium, the authors concluded that calcium was preferentially absorbed by the fetal gut. Kopito and Shwachman (1966) estimated the concentration of sodium, potassium, calcium, magnesium, phosphorous, copper, zinc, manganese and iron in meconium from healthy neonates and infants with cystic fibrosis. Although the mean values of all the ion concentrations were lower in meconium from cystic fibrosis infants, the variances were so great that the differences between the mean values were not statistically signficant. The total contribution of these ions is 1–2% of the total dry weight.

18

Haemoglobin Metabolites

Haemoglobin metabolites present in meconium reflect the result of gut metabolism free of intestinal flora. Apart from the bile pigments such as bilirubin which are responsible for the intense colour of meconium, four porphyrins have been detected (French & Thonger, 1966). The main porphyrin is coproporphyrin I, with trace amounts of protoporphyrin and two others, characterised by their spectra. One of these porphyrins, designated porphyrin S411, has recently been characterised by French and colleagues (1972) as a monacylic derivative of coproporphyrin III.

Steroids

Over 30 steroids have been characterised in meconium, usually in very small amounts (Gustafasson & Stenberg, 1971; Kinsella & Francis, 1971). They are mainly metabolites of various steroid hormones and are present as mono and disulphate derivatives. Their main source of origin is not clear. Bile acids, C_{24} steroid derivatives, have been reported to be present in unexpectedly low concentrations, 20 μg per gram dry weight (Miettinen & Luukkainen, 1968).

Sterols

The major sterols present in meconium are cholesterol and lathosterol in ester and unesterfied forms and more than five other sterols have been characterised (Miettinen & Luukkainen, 1968; Eneroth, et al, 1969). It has been suggested that much of the sterols in meconium originate from the vernix caseosa (Miettinen & Luukkainen, 1968).

MECONIUM COMPOSITION IN DISEASE

As the composition of meconium from healthy neonates is at least partially established, it should be possible to detect changes due to underlying pathological disorders with particular emphasis on the fetal gut. The detection of such changes would not only provide useful information about the biochemical nature of such disorders but would also provide an early diagnosis of disease in the newborn. To date, such changes in composition have only been studied in detail with respect to cystic fibrosis. Several workers have suggested other possible changes in meconium composition which could be related to the underlying gut pathology but such suggestions still need to be fully investigated.

Cystic Fibrosis

Cystic fibrosis is one of the most common of the genetic inherited diseases with an incidence of one in 2,000 births in Europe and North America. It is manifested

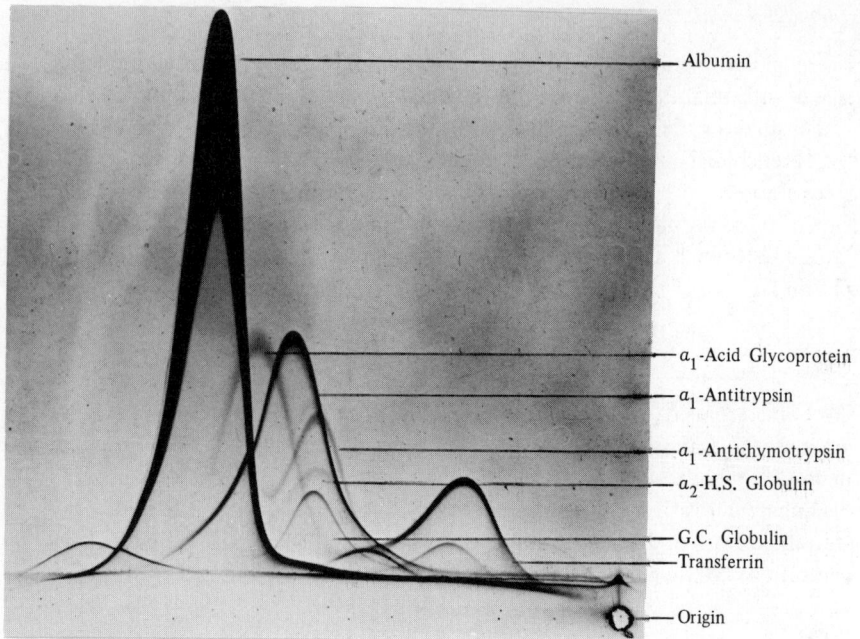

Figure 2. Crossed immunoelectrophoretic pattern of meconium from an infant with cystic fibrosis against rabbit antihuman serum. Electrophoresis and staining were carried out by methods previously described (Ryley et al, 1974). The elevated protein content in meconium from cystic fibrosis infants can be seen to be due not only to an increased albumin concentration but also due to an increase in the number of other serum proteins present.

by a systemic disorder of the mucous glands resulting in hypersecretion of epithelial mucus. Aspects of cystic fibrosis have recently been reviewed by Talmo and Austin (1972); Polley and Bearn (1974). About 80% of infants with cystic fibrosis suffer from insufficiency of secreted pancreatic proteolytic activity and meconium ileus is associated with 10–15% of such infants. The most significant effect on the composition of meconium, where pancreatic insufficiency is present, is a marked elevation of protein content; first reported in meconium ileus patients (Glanzmann & Berger, 1950; Rapoport & Buchanan, 1950) and also found in meconium from neonates with cystic fibrosis but without symptoms of meconium ileus (Wiser & Beier, 1964). Green, et al (1958) demonstrated that most of the protein was albumin but numerous other serum proteins may also be identified in meconium from infants with cystic fibrosis (Ryley et al, 1974)–Figure 2. It has been suggested that a simple screening method for cystic fibrosis may be developed which depends on a test for protein in meconium (Green et al, 1958; Wiser & Beier, 1964; Hobbs, 1969; Stephan et al, 1975; Kollberg & Hellsing, 1975) but unfortunately such tests give a 0.5–1.0% false positive result, and more important, false negative results have also been reported (Prosser et al, 1974; Ryley, et al, 1975).

Another approach for the detection of cystic fibrosis by the analysis of meconium would be to determine differences in the composition and distribution of the mucins. With so little known about the mucins of meconium, opinion, based on analysis of duodenal fluids from older children, is divided as to whether or not there are differences in structure and composition of gut mucins in cystic fibrosis (Schultze & Heremans, 1966; di Sant'Agnese & Talamo, 1967) and an answer to the problem is still awaited.

Other Diseases of the Gut

Other diseases than cystic fibrosis such as hereditary pancreatic insufficiency with chronic neutropenia, congenital atresia of the pancreatic duct and trypsinogen deficiency disease are characterised by a lack of pancreatic proteolytic activity and thus meconium from infants suffering from these diseases should also contain elevated protein content (Hobbs, 1969).

Conversely, infants with oesophageal atresia without a fistula have a marked absence of even the protease inhibitors in their meconium (Ryley, unpublished). It is suggested that an absence of α_1-antitrypsin but not α_1-antichymotrypsin indicates a deficiency of this anti-protease in the amniotic fluid and hence in the maternal vascular system (Ryley et al, 1975). Such an infant should be screened for α_1-antitrypsin deficiency as an infant with α_1-antitrypsin deficiency would be at risk of developing neonatal hepatitis (Talmo & Austin, 1972).

Disaccharidase deficiency often leads to clinical disaccharide intolerance. Eggermont (1966) has suggested that meconium from infants at risk should be screened for the presence of these enzymes in their meconium. Although a negative result would not be conclusive evidence for possible glycosidase deficiency, a positive result would be strong evidence against the possible development of disaccharide intolerance.

Bile pigment deficiency resulting in a grey or yellow meconium stool is a sign of congenital bile duct atresia (Windle, 1971) although this is not invariably the case. Fashena (1948) reported that there is an inverse relationship between bile pigment content of meconium and the subsequent development of neonatal hyperbilirubinaemia.

CONCLUSIONS

It would be unwise to draw any conclusions concerning the biochemistry of the developing fetal gut based solely on evidence of meconium composition. Not only are the potential sources of many of the components extremely diverse but marked changes occur to the fetal gut contents prior to and during agglomeration into the

21

final meconial mass. A knowledge of the composition of meconium is of more use when comparing specimens from healthy infants with specimens from infants with alimentary tract disorders. Changes revealed by such a comparison may increase our understanding of the underlying pathology of diseases that affect the neonatal gut and, perhaps more important, detection of such changes may provide a useful diagnostic aid for disease in the newborn well before outward clinical signs are manifested. At the moment, apart from changes caused by cystic fibrosis, this aspect of the biochemistry of meconium has been largely neglected.

References

Andersen, H, Bierring, F, Matthiessen, M, Egeberg, J and Bro-Rasmussen, F (1964) *Acta Pathologica et Microbioligica Scandinavica, 61,* 377

Becker, R F, Windle, W F, Barth, E E and Schultz, M D (1940) *Surgery, Gynecology and Obstetrics, 70,* 603

Buchanan, D J and Rapoport, S (1951) *Journal of Biological Chemistry, 192,* 251

di Sant'Agnese, P A and Talamo, R C (1968) *New England Journal of Medicine, 277,* 1287

Eggermont, E (1966) *Biology of the Neonate, 10,* 266

Eneroth, P, Gustafasson, J A and Nystrom, E (1969) *European Journal of Biochemistry, 11,* 456

Fashena, G J (1948) *American Journal of Diseases of Children, 76,* 196

Fraser, D and Clamp, J R (1975) *Clinica Chimica Acta, 59,* 301

French, J M and Thonger, E (1966) *Clinical Science, 31,* 337

French, J M, Nicholson, D C and Rimington, C (1970) *Biochemical Journal, 120,* 393

Glanzmann, E and Berger, H (1950) *Annales paediatrici, 175,* 33

Green, M N, Clarke, J T and Shwachman, H (1958) *Pediatrics, 21,* 635

Gustafasson, J A and Stenberg, A (1971) *European Journal of Biochemistry, 22,* 246

Hall, I C and O'Toole, E (1934) *American Journal of Diseases of Children, 47,* 1279

Hobbs, J R (1969) *Protides of Biological Fluids, 16,* 517

Kimura, A and Nagai, T (1964) *Fukushima Journal of Medical Science, 11,* 59

Kinsella, R A and Francis, F E (1971) *Journal of Clinical Endocrinology and Metabolism, 32,* 801

Kollberg, H and Hellsing, K (1975) *Acta Paediatrica Scandinavica, 64,* 477

Kopito, L and Shwachman, H (1966) *Journal of Pediatrics, 68,* 313

Miettinen, T A and Luukkainen, T (1968) *Acta Chemica Scandinavica, 22,* 2603

Polley, M J and Bearn, A G (1974) *Journal of Medical Genetics, 11,* 249

Pritchard, J A (1966) *Obstetrics and Gynecology, 28,* 606

Prosser, R, Owen, H, Bull, F, Parry, B, Smerkinich, J, Goodwin, H A and Dathan, J (1974), *Archives of Disease in Childhood, 49,* 597

Rapoport, S and Buchanan, D J (1950) *Science, 112,* 150

Roulet, D L A and von Muralt, G (1961) *Schweizerische Medizinische Wochenschrift, 91,* 74

Rule, A H and Goleski-Reilly, C (1973) *Immunological Communications, 2,* 213

Ryley, H C (1972) *Biochemical Journal, 128,* 129P

Ryley, H C, Neale, M L, Brogan, T D and Bray, P T (1974) *Archives of Disease in Childhood, 49,* 901

Ryley, H C, Neale, M L, Brogan, T D and Bray, P T (1975) *Clinica Chimica Acta* (in press)

Schachter, H and Dixon, G H (1965) *Canadian Journal of Biochemistry, 43,* 381

Schultze, H E and Heremans, J F (1966) *Molecular Biology of Human Proteins, Vol. I* Elsevier Publishing Company, Amsterdam. Pages 547–556, and 796–798.

Schwarz, E (1953) *Annales paediatrici, 181,* 306

Schwidt, W (1971) *Verhanlungen Anatomischen Gesellschaft, 66,* 55

Smith, C A (1959) *The Physiology of the Newborn Infant, 3rd ed.* Blackwell, Oxford. Pages 235–250

Stephan, U, Busch, E W, Hellsing, K and Kollberg, H (1975) *Pediatrics, 55,* 35
Talmo, R C and Austin, K F (1972) *Bronchopulmonary Disease and Related Disorders,*
  Vol. I. (Ed Holman, C W and Muschenhein, C.) Harper and Row, New York, Pages 167–178
Widdowson, E M, McCance, R A, Harrison, G E and Sutton, A (1962) *Lancet, ii,* 373
Windle, W F (1971) *Physiology of the Fetus,* C. C. Thomas, Springfield. Pages 94–100
Wiser, W C and Beier, F R (1964) *Pediatrics, 33,* 115

Discussion

MR FREEMAN   Dr Ryley, I am interested in meconium from a surgeon's point of view and I would like to ask some questions. First, whether you accept that the baby does not pass meconium in utero under normal conditions?

DR RYLEY   I must say straight away, I am a biochemist not a clinician, but I understand this is so, yes, except in fetal distress.

FREEMAN   It raises an interesting point: why in babies with rectal atresia do you see an enormous accumulation of meconium in the colon above the atresia?

RYLEY   I don't know.

FREEMAN   Have you had an opportunity to study the meconium plug syndrome?

RYLEY   No, we have not.

DR LITTLEWOOD   In how many babies during a screening for cystic fibrosis have you found a positive albumin in the meconium, and secondly, have these babies been looked at and followed up clinically?

RYLEY   It depends what you define as a positive albumin.

LITTLEWOOD   Say 20 mg.

RYLEY   We have had 9 out of about 5,000 tested, who were followed up and were apparently normal, and the rest had cystic fibrosis. On the other hand, three of the infants who were shown on sweat test at least to have cystic fibrosis had albumin contents of 10 mg and less. So we normally now screen for albumin as low as 5 mg. There is a higher proportion of positive results in infants who are premature. About 5% of all infants would need to be screened by sweat tests, but we do have a plan to increase efficiency of tests on meconium for pancreatic insufficiency as well as presence of protein, which would improve our discrimination and avoid this large number of sweat tests.

LITTLEWOOD   How long are they followed through? Do you know that the test indicates the presence of a form of pancreatic insufficiency, as was suggested?

RYLEY   We compare a protein which is liable to proteolysis, albumin, with a protein which is resistant to proteolysis, antitrypsin. When you look at the ratio, if there was complete absence of proteolytic activity, then one would expect the ratio to be 10, that is, there would be 10 times as much albumin. Now we find that this ratio in cystic fibrosis, where the albumin is high, is about 6, so that there is probably a little proteolytic activity but not enough to affect the albumin concentration to any great extent. Now, we would follow up any child, no matter what this ratio was, where the albumin content was about 20 mg. We found that this ratio dropped to less than 0.1 within three days in all cases of the nine normals that we studied. In cystic fibrosis this is not so, the ratio is maintained at the high value. Of course, in pancreatic enzyme deficiency diseases not related to cystic fibrosis, one would expect the same thing to happen, but we have not had a negative sweat test with the maintenance of apparent pancreatic insufficiency.

PROFESSOR HADORN   I think it is very important that Dr Ryley examined this in great detail. Those of us who have an interest in cystic fibrosis have heard about the co-ordinated study which is going on in Europe. Dr Stephan has collected the results, and I believe 13% were negative, out of 150,000 meconium tests done. The expected frequency of the children with cystic fibrosis detected by the sweat test would be around 1 in 1,500, and it was very interesting to see that Stephan with his screening method found a frequency of 1 in 1,650. This is therefore according to these screening data the frequency of cystic fibrosis in Europe, but, of course, many cases have been missed with albumin tests and these are the cases who will be shown in the future to have cystic fibrosis, although they have no early manifestation. There is still a large correction to be made.

RYLEY   I would say our figure, based on a very small series, was even higher: 3 negatives for meconium protein out of 19 cystics diagnosed. In fact, two of the three were sibs, and one was picked up pretty soon after birth, because it is automatic to do sweat tests on sibs of known patients.

DR PROSSER   I think the 'false negative' figure for Wales is 30%, and this is of course higher than Stephan expected.

RYLEY   This is of course with the Boehringer Meconium test, which needs 20 mg of albumin to give a positive result.

24

HADORN   We have always tried to make sure that those cases who were negative were all studied, because some of them might have normal pancreatic functions, but, unfortunately, this has not been done, or only in very few cases. We had a case in Bern where we found the meconium albumin test to be negative and the child was then found to have cystic fibrosis in a very severe pulmonary form. The child died soon and came to autopsy, and I also investigated pancreatic function by secretory tests. I found a normal pancreatic function, and this was corroborated by post mortem findings of a completely normal pancreas. So we are absolutely in agreement with the idea that those with a normal pancreas will digest their albumin but will not digest the α-1 antitrypsin and therefore I think that this ratio, if it could be done systematically, would perhaps be the answer.

RYLEY   We found in all three cases with a negative result in meconium, that within three months this ratio had risen to above three in the faeces. One is by this time dealing with alpha-1 antitrypsin which is present due to purely passive transudation. In meconium the albumin values in cystics are perhaps 200 mg/g dry weight compared to zero for normals. In the faeces they are something like 2 mg compared with zero and therefore this ratio does help to highlight the development of absence of gut protelytic enzyme.

25

Origin and Development of the Rodent Gastrointestinal Pancreatic Tract Endocrine Cells

JULIA M POLAK, A G E PEARSE, MARIANNE VAN MOURIK and MARION L GRAY

Summary

The development of the endocrine cells of the gut and pancreas in mice can be divided into three stages:

day 9 to day 14: numerous 'clear' cells can be seen in the primitive gut and some in the pancreatic rudiment. Ultrastructural studies show the presence of scattered primitive secretory granules which have a limiting membrane and are polymorphic;

day 14 to day 16: an intermediate stage, characterised by the more mature appearance of the secretory granules, further development of the gut (upper-mid and low) and of the pancreatic rudiment (ductular and acinar formation) and appearance, at day 15.5 onwards, of some immunocytochemical reactions to gastrointestinal pancreatic hormones;

day 16 onwards: the gut and pancreas are fully developed. Histological stains for secretory granules are positive as well as immunocytochemical stains for gut hormones. The electron-dense secretory granules have all the morphological characteristics at the ultrastructural level which appear in the adult (Wiesbaden classification). Quantitative immunocytochemistry of the gastrointestinal hormones reveals that the hormonal pattern, present in the adult, is already present in embryo.

It is postulated that the neuroectodermal cells of the neural crest may be the precursor of some or all of the endocrine cells of the gastrointestinal pancreatic system.

The existence of endocrine cells in the gastrointestinal mucosa was first suggested by Masson as early as 1914. In 1938 Feyrter described his diffuse 'endokrine Organe', a system of clear cells (Helle Zellen) which were distributed throughout the body either in discrete organs or as single elements among non-endocrine

26

cells. Feyrter's (1938, 1953) studies of this system were based on three characteristics shown by his 'clear' cells:
1) Clarity (emptiness of the cytoplasm in conventionally stained preparations).
2) Argentaffinity (ability to reduce silver solutions).
3) Argyrophilia (ability to take up and retain silver salts which can subsequently be reduced by chemical methods.)

Since the 1960s it has become clear that the cells responsible for the production of peptide hormones have certain histological and ultrastructural characteristics which have been thoroughly investigated and described by a number of workers (Carvalheira et al, 1968; Orci et al, 1968; Solcia et al, 1968; Forssman et al, 1969; Solcia et al, 1969; Forssman, 1970; Kobayashi et al, 1970; Sasagawa et al, 1970; Solcia et al, 1970; Osaka et al, 1971; Fujita, 1973; and many others).

These cells can also be identified by certain more specific cytochemical and functional properties and have been grouped together as the APUD cell series (Pearse, 1968, 1969). The two most characteristic properties of the APUD cells are firstly the production and storage of various types of amines and, secondly, the production of low molecular weight peptides which may or may not be proven hormones in the strict physiological sense (Pearse, 1966a and b; 1968, 1969). The APUD (Amine or amine Precursor Uptake and Decarboxylation) series now has more than 30 members.

According to the APUD concept all the constituent endocrine peptide-producing cells of the series are to be considered as derivatives of neural ectoderm (Pearse 1966a and b). Embryological evidence supporting the postulated neuro-ectodermal origin of the APUD cells comes from many sources. Studies using a quail/chick allograft technique, with the use of a biological marker system to identify donor cells in the resulting chimeras (Le Douarin, 1969) have provided complete validation in the case of the ultimobranchial C cells (Le Douarin & Le Lièvre, 1971), and the type I cells of the carotid body (Le Douarin et al, 1972). Cytochemical marker experiments (Pearse & Polak, 1971a; Polak et al, 1971; Pearse, Polak et al, 1973) have provided confirmation for these biological marker studies and also, in combination with the work of Pearse and Carvalheira (1967), for the thyroid C cells. *Total* proof of the production of a 'peripheral' peptide hormone (calcitonin) by the cells of neural crest origin has been obtained only in the case of the avian ultimobranchial gland. This was achieved by combining the biological marker technique with sequential immunocyto-chemistry (Polak et al, 1974).

In the case of the endocrine cells of the gut and pancreas, cytochemical marker experiments, using both avian and rodent embryos, have provided circumstantial evidence in favour of a neuroectodermal origin (Pearse & Polak, 1971b; Pearse et al, 1973). Although much is known about the endocrine cells of both gut and pancreas, there is only sketchy information on their development. In the gut of avian and rodent embryos the morphogenesis of argentaffin and argyrophil cells has been described (Kull, 1913-1925; Parat, 1924; Cordier, 1926; Simard & Campenhout, 1932; Sharples, 1945; Monesi, 1960; Penttilä, 1968; Larsson et al, 1975). The endocrine pancreas has received more attention. Numerous and extensive studies on various aspects of the development of the mammalian endocrine pancreas have been made since the pioneer work of Laguesse (1869). These studies (e.g. Hard, 1944; McAlpine, 1951; Ferreira, 1957; Frye, 1957; Munger, 1958; Esterhuizen, 1959; Golosow & Grobstein, 1962; Grillo, 1964; Hellman, 1965-66; Pictet et al, 1968; Wessells & Rutter, 1969; Perrier, 1970; Spooner et al, 1970; Pictet et al, 1971) have produced a mass of controversial findings.

The work reported here comprises the application of immunocytochemical and ultrastructural techniques to the development of the endocrine cells of the pancreas and gut of the rodent embryo.

Material and methods

Seventy-two embryos, from 11 pregnant CSI albino mice were studied. Gestation was terminated at periods from the 10th to the 19th day and the age of each embryo was verified from the external features using criteria established by Gruneberg (1943). Where possible (from 14 days onwards) the pancreas and gut were dissected out and the gut was then subdivided into three regions (upper-mid-lower). Earlier embryos were frozen and processed whole (10-14 days).

Light microscopy

The whole embryos (up to 14 days) or blocks from the dissected gut or pancreas were immediately quenched in Arcton (Freon) at −156°C and freeze-dried in a thermo-electric freeze-drier. Subsequently the blocks were vapour fixed in DEPC (diethylpyrocarbonate) or *p*-benzoquinone for 3 hours at 60°C (Pearse et al, 1974; Pearse & Polak, 1975) and then embedded in paraffin wax. 5μm sections were stained with haematoxylin-eosin in order to check the orientation of the block and preservation of the tissue. An indirect (sandwich) method for immuno-histochemistry (Coons et al, 1955) was then carried out using antibodies to the following peptides: gastrin (Polak et al, 1972); GIP [gastric inhibitory poly-peptide] (Polak et al, 1973); glucagon and insulin (Pearse et al, 1973); VIP [Vasoactive intestinal polypeptide] (Polak et al, 1974); EG (Enteroglucagon) (Polak et al, 1971), and secretin (Polak et al, 1971). Immunofluorescent preparations were viewed in a Leitz Orthoplan microscope fitted with HBO 100 and XBO 75 lamps and a Ploem illuminator. the FITC labelled sections were excited at 490 nm using two KP 490 interference filters and a TK 510 dichroic mirror. A K 515 filter barrier was employed and photomicrographs were taken on Ilford FP 4 film.

Quantitative Immunocytochemistry

One hundred and fifty 5μm sections were cut from each block, for quantitative immunocytochemistry. Five sections were taken at intervals of 30 sections from every region of the gut and immunoperoxidase staining was carried out with the antibodies to the gut hormones referred to above. Quantification was carried out with the Quantimet 720 D. This instrument is a combined microscope and scanning integrating image analyser capable of measuring both the absorption of light by a tissue section component, and the total area in which this absorption occurs. It can thus provide quantitative measurement of the product of a histochemical reaction. The microscopic field is scanned and the image is converted to an electronic signal which is then analysed. Using this instrument we have been able to obtain information as to the number of endocrine cells per unit area.

Electron Microscopy

Blocks from younger embryos containing gut and/or pancreas, and small pieces of the gut and pancreas from older animals, were fixed in 3% glutaraldehyde in 0.1 M phosphate buffer (pH 7.2) for at least 3 hours. After fixation the tissues were washed out for 2 hours in several changes of 0.01 M phosphate buffer (pH 7.2) containing 0.1 M sucrose. They were then post-fixed in 1% osmium tetroxide in Millonig's buffer (pH 7.0) for one hour. After dehydration in ascending grades of ethyl alcohol, and two changes of propylene oxide, the blocks were left overnight at 45° in a mixture of Araldite resin, hardener and dibutyl-phthalate. They were then embedded in Araldite mixture with BMDA (benzyl diemthylamine) accelerator and polymerised at 60°C. The blocks from the younger embryos were embedded flat in polythene embedding trays and the others in capsules in the usual manner.

Blocks from whole embryos were trimmed on an LKB Pyramitome until the desired area was reached. This was found by staining 2μm sections with toluidine blue in 3% borax. The blocks were then trimmed to a pyramid containing the area to be examined and ultrathin sections were cut on a Cambridge Huxley ultramicrotome. Sections from older embryos were also cut on this instrument. All sections were stained with 15% uranyl acetate in methanol, followed by lead citrate. They were viewed in an AEI EM 6B microscope.

Results

The development of the endocrine cells of the gut and pancreas was considered in three stages, the first from day 10 to 14, the second from day 14 to 16 and the third from day 16 onwards (see Table I).

TABLE I. Development of the Endocrine Cells of the Rodent Gastrointestinal Pancreatic Tract

	Conventional Stains	Methods for endocrine granules	APUD–FIF	Immunocytochemistry	Ultrastructure
10–14 days	Clear cells among other epithelial cells. Formation of dorsal pancreas.	Negative	Positive	Negative	Endocrine cells of a single type (13–14 days). Pleomorphic, with moderately electron-dense secretory granules.
14–16 days	Gut further developed into foregut, mid-gut and hind-gut. Dorsal and ventral pancreas with islet formation.	Negative except for argentaffinity(+)	Positive, and also FIF alone in EC cells.	Positive on or just before the 16th day.	Further non-endocrine differentiation (zymogen granules and mucin). Endocrine cells with primitive and more differentiated type of granules (transitional forms).
16th day onwards	Gradual development of all the features found in adult mice	Positive (towards the end of the gestational period).	Strongly positive APUD–FIF and FIF.	Strongly positive for all hormones.	Presence of well differentiated endocrine cells with granules of all (Wiesbaden) types.

Day 10 to day 14

Sections of the primitive gut, conventionally stained with haematoxylin and eosin or toluidine blue, showed numerous clear cells amongst the epithelial cells of the intestinal wall (Figure 1). Electron microscopy at this stage revealed endocrine cells of a single type (Figure 2) containing pleomorphic, moderately electron-dense, granules.

Formation of the dorsal pancreas was observed to begin at about the 11th day with the bulging outwards of a group of cells in the upper wall of the intestine. This bulge gave rise to a plumb diverticulum which was closely apposed to and surrounded by condensed mesenchyme. At this stage all the specific stains for secretory granules were negative, as was immunocytochemistry of all the hormones investigated.

However, as has already been reported, the APUD (Pearse et al, 1973) characteristics of the primitive endocrine cells were readily demonstrable after injection of *L*-DOPA into the mother.

At the electron microscope level the undifferentiated cells of the pancreatic rudiment were seen to be round or oval in shape, with dense cytoplasm containing numerous free ribosomes. Some of the cells contained secretion granules of endocrine type, similar to those described above.

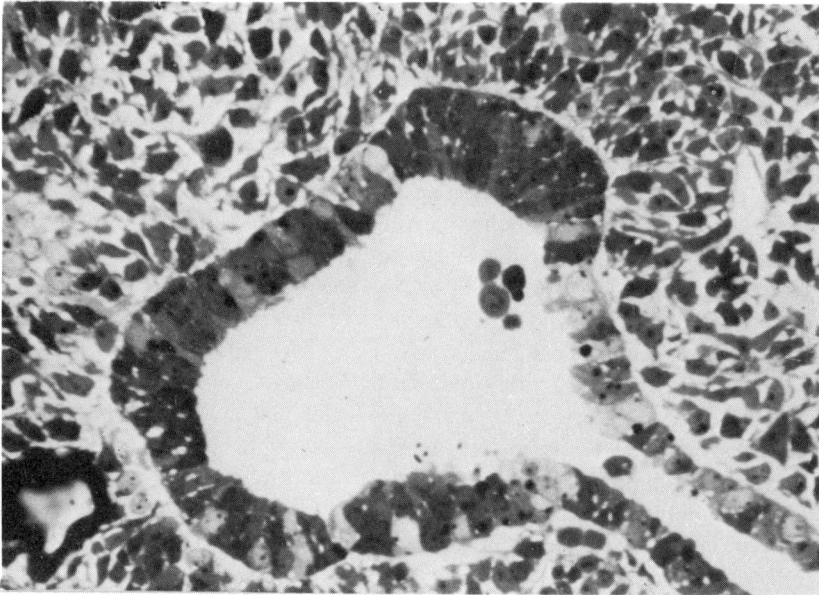

Figure 1. 11 day-old mouse embryo. Resin embedded. Mid-gut area showing numerous 'clear' cells in between epithelial non-endocrine elements. Toluidine blue   X 344

31

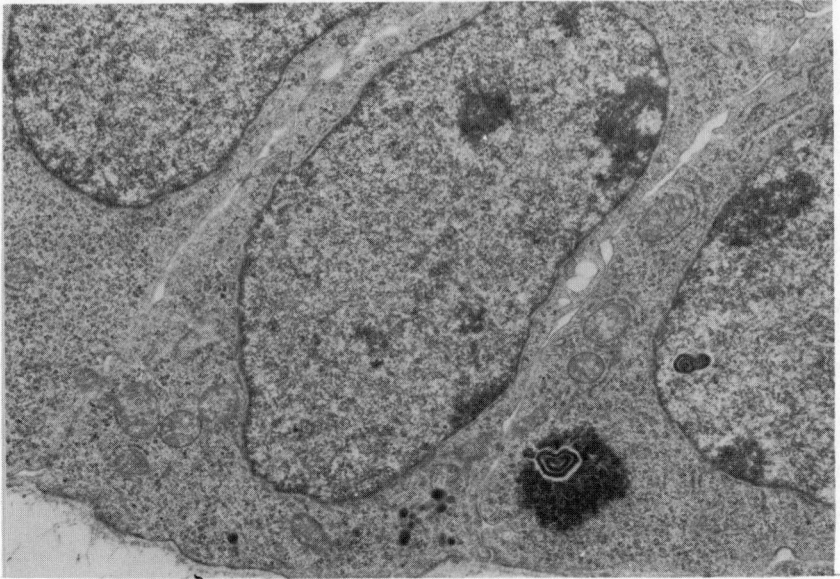

Figure 2. 11 day-old mouse embryo. Ultrastructural appearance of the primitive endocrine secretory granules characteristic of stage 1 (10—14 days).   X 14.500

Day 14 to 16

At this stage the gut is further developed into foregut, midgut and hindgut. The epithelial non-endocrine cells show signs of differentiation towards mucin production and the endocrine cells (clear cells) can now be stained by argentaffin methods (Pearse et al, 1973). Other specific histological methods for endocrine granules are still negative or only weakly positive. Immunocytochemical reactions for nearly all the hormones become weakly positive by the end of this period. The pancreatic rudiment is observed to grow continuously. Optical microscopy revealed numerous branching cords of primitive cells with occasional glandular lumina. Ultrastructural studies showed a higher proportion of cells containing endocrine-type secretion granules which had an increased electron density and a visible limiting membrane, sometimes with a halo in addition. Intermediate forms could be seen between the primitive undifferentiated granule (Figure 3) and the more mature forms, which could sometimes be recognised as one of the endocrine types of the Wiesbaden classification (Creutzfeldt et al, 1969).

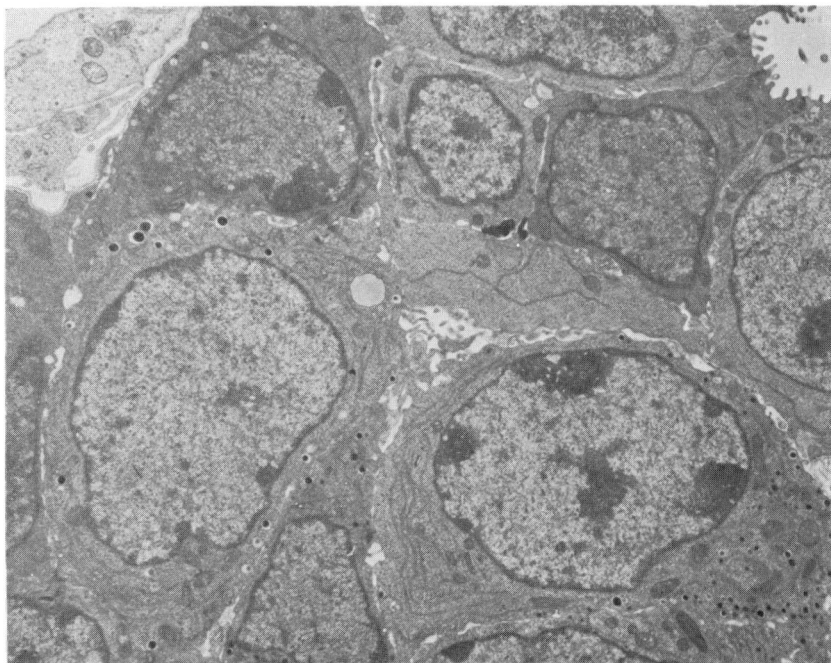

Figure 3. 15 day-old mouse embryo. Secretory granules with intermediate forms. × 7000

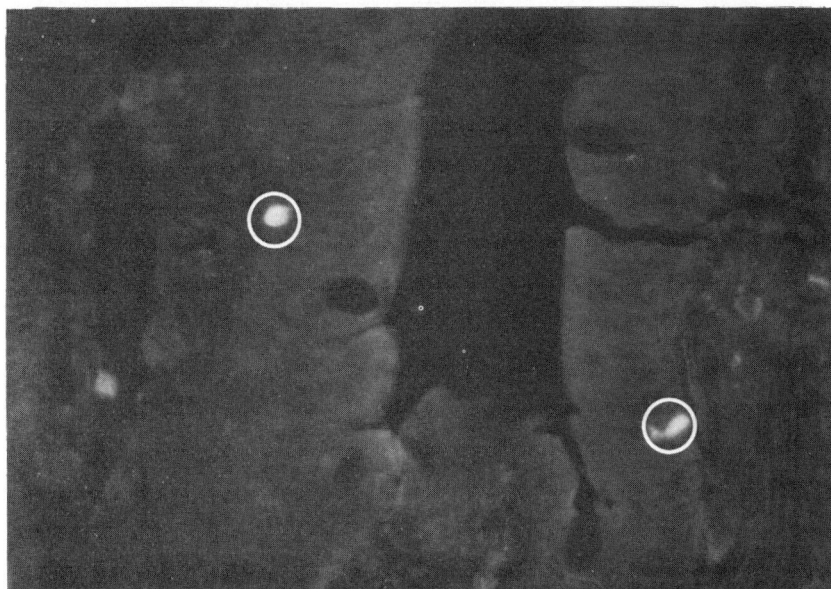

Figure 4. 19 day-old mouse embryo. Gut mucosa stained with antibodies to gastrin. Two positive cells can be seen.　　　× 344

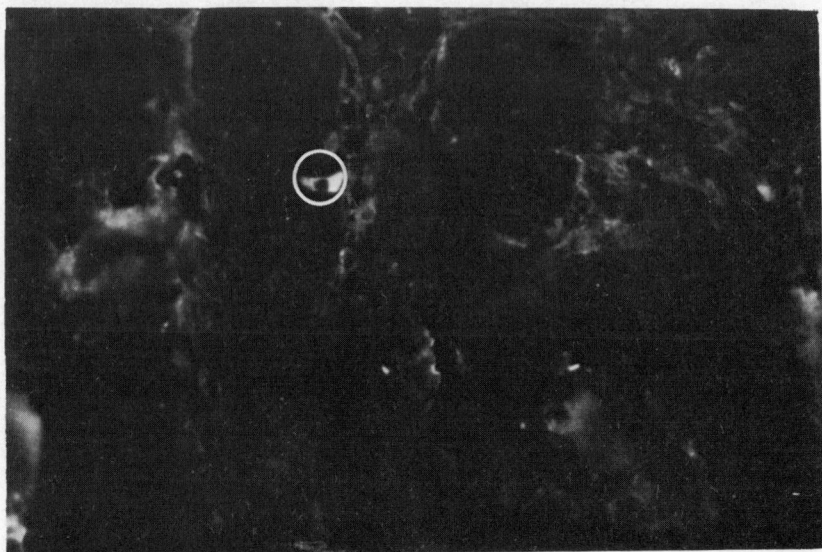

Figure 5. 19 day-old mouse embryo. Gut mucosa stained with antibodies to secretin. A positive cell can be seen in one of the glands. X 344

16 days onwards

At this stage both histological and immunocytochemical stains for secretion granules are positive and become stronger towards the end of the gestational period (Figures 4, 5). Ultrastructural studies indicate a possible differentiation between various types of endocrine cells responsible for the production of the various peptide hormones (Figure 6).

Quantitative Studies of the Gut Endocrine Cells

Antral gastrin-producing cells are seen first at 15.5 days. The number of cells per unit are increased in the first few days, decreased in the days following, and increased again just before birth (Figure 7).

The number of gastrin-immunoreactive cells in the embryonic intestine corresponds to the pattern of the adult (greater concentrations in the upper or mid-intestine). There is a small increase in the number of cells at 17 days, but this is not highly significant. It is important to note that the number of positive cells present in the lower intestine increased with age, and this discrepancy with the upper intestine indicates that we are probably dealing not only with gastrin cells but also with cells producing cholecystokinin (CCK). This peptide cross reacts with antibodies to the C-terminal portion of gastrin (Figure 8).

34

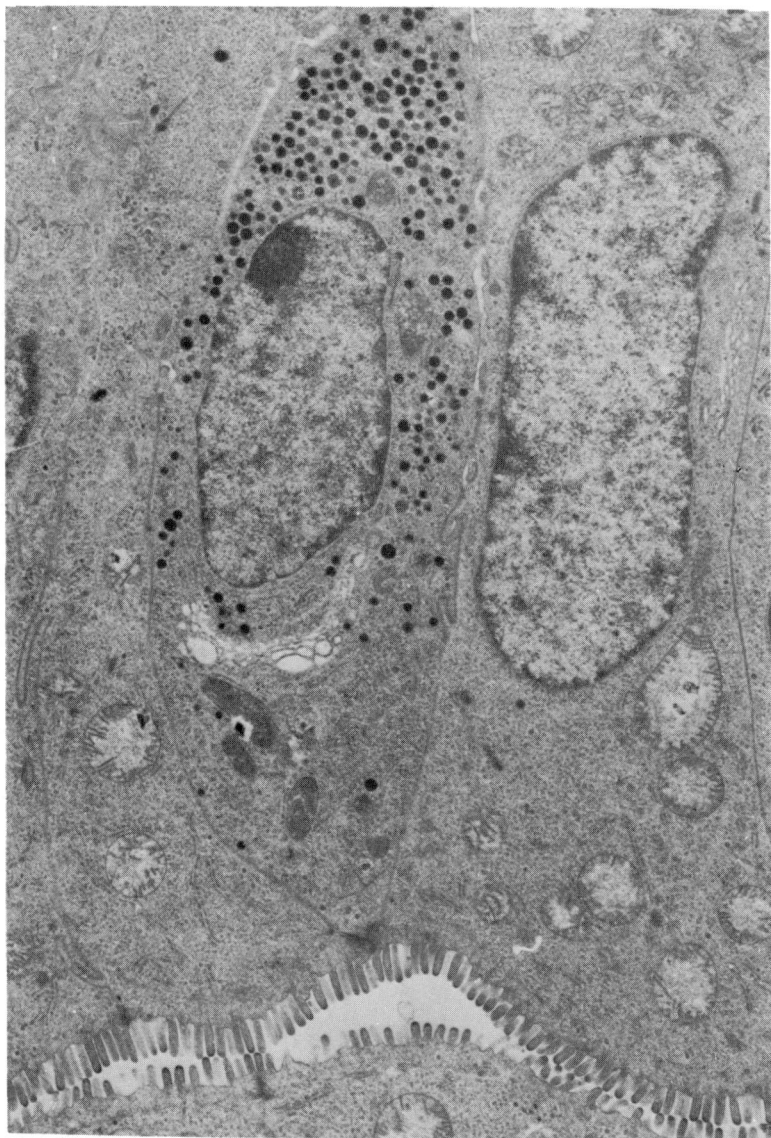

Figure 6. 18 day-old mouse embryo. Ultrastructurally identifiable endocrine cell of the midgut. Note the presence of numerous electron-dense secretory granules on the basal part of the cell and its connection with the intestinal lumen through a tuft of microvilli.

x 7.500

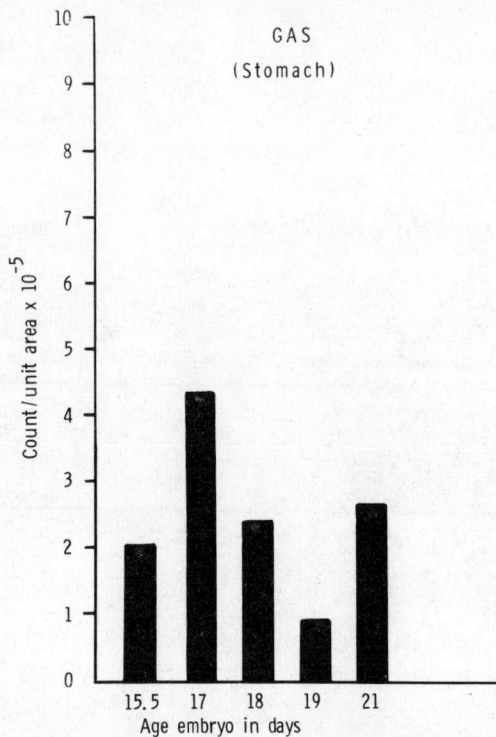

Figure 7. Number of antral G cell/per unit area at various stages of the embryonic life.

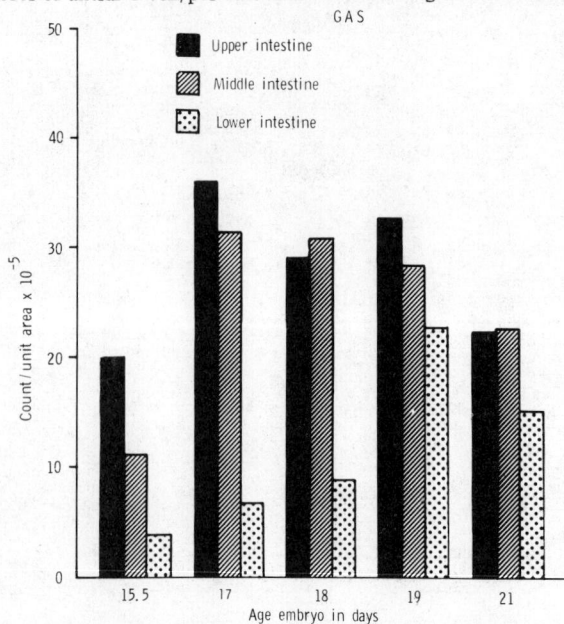

Figure 8. Number of intestinal gastrin-immunoreactive cells/per unit area and its relationship with the age of the embryo.

36

The distribution pattern of GIP cells, judging by the number of cells per unit, is also similar to that found in the adult, with, again, a small peak of higher concentration in the upper intestine at 17 days (Figure 9). Secretin-producing cells are mostly concentrated in the upper and mid-intestine. The peak number of cells per unit area, unlike that of the other hormones described above, appears at 19 days (Figure 10). VIP cells per unit area are randomly distributed in the three areas of the embryonic intestine while in the adult they are chiefly found in the lower intestine (Figure 11). Enteroglucagon cells on the other hand seem to be distributed as in the adult, with the exception of a peak in the upper intestine at 19 days (Figure 12).

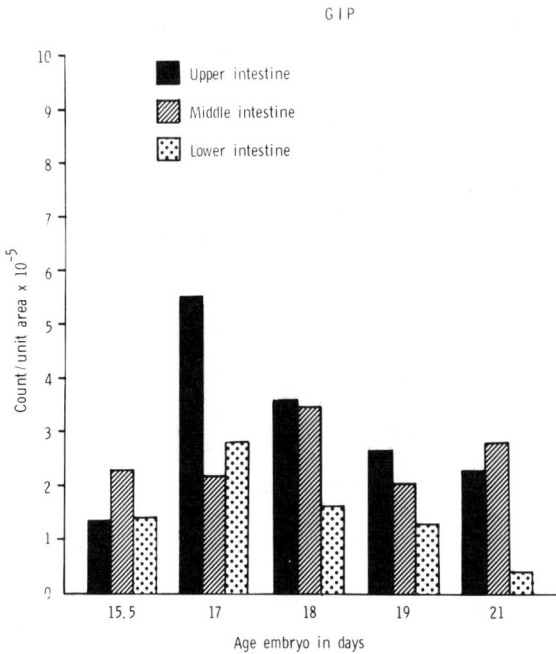

Figure 9. Quantitative immunocytochemistry for GIP cells in the embryonic intestine (various ages).

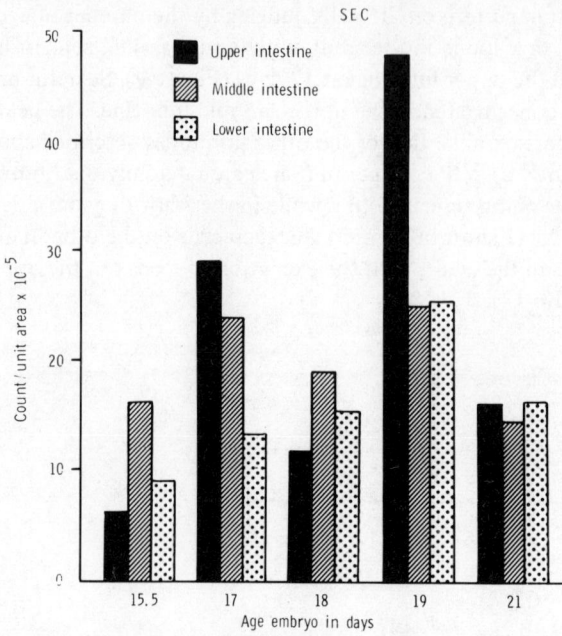

Figure 10. The number of secretin producing cells/per unit are in various parts of the embryonic intestine is similar to that of adult ratio.

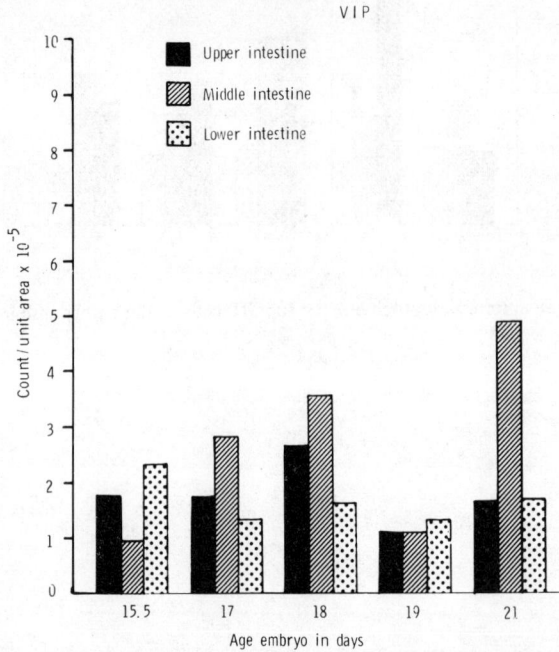

Figure 11. Number of VIP producing cells/per unit area in various parts of the embryonic gut.

38

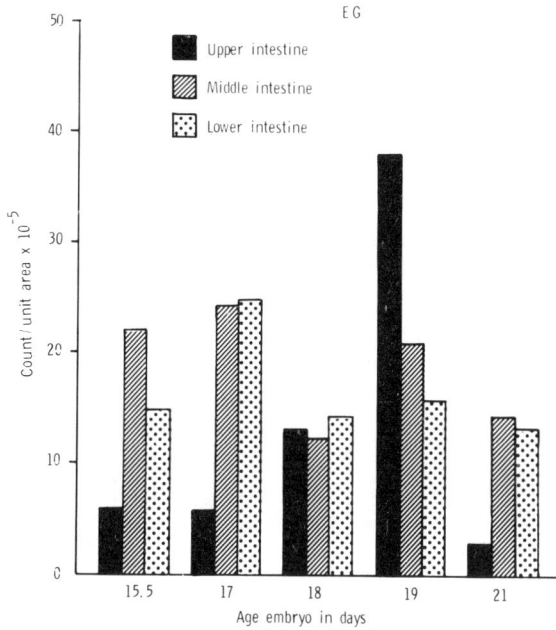

Figure 12. Number of EG cells/per unit area in various parts of the embryonic gut.

Discussion

We have followed the development and differentiation of the endocrine cells of the gut and pancreas from an early stage up to the time of birth. With regard to the development of the islet cells, our results can be compared to those of other workers in the field (see Table in Pearse, et al, 1973). On the other hand there are very few studies with which to compare our results on the gut endocrine cells. We have found that well differentiated endocrine cells appear first at 15.5 days in the mouse embryo. Monesi (1960) found argentaffin cells in the chick embryo at 15.5—16 days of incubation and his findings agree with those of Kull (1913-1925) and Cordier (1926), whereas Simard and Campenhout (1932) record the earliest appearance at 10—11 days. In rat embryos the first appearance of argentaffin cells was recorded between 15—17 days (Sharples, 1945) and in sheep, cat, dog, guinea-pig and horse, towards the end of the intrauterine life (Parat, 1924a). Using the technique of formaldehyde induced fluorescence (Eränkö, 1955a, 1967; Falck & Torp, 1961; Penttilä, 1968) Eränkö records the first appearance of amine-containing cells in the gut epithelium at 13.5 to 14 days in the chick embryo.

39

It is important to note that in general terms the distribution of hormones in the gastrointestinal mucosa, as estimated by quantitative immunocytochemistry, agrees with the distribution of these hormones in adults (Bloom et al, 1975). The variable peak of higher numbers which appears at some stages of the development, should be regarded as due to a disproportionate rate of development between the gut mucosa and the endocrine cells. The previously reported formaldehyde-induced fluorescence (Pearse et al, 1973), and the finding in this study of a common type of ultrastructurally identifiable primitive secretory granule in both gut and pancreas, was regarded as evidence supporting a common neuroectodermal origin for the cells of the APUD series (Pearse & Takor Takor, 1975). *A priori* there are three developmental possibilities for the (clear) cells with APUD—FIF characteristics and primitive secretory granules:

1) They arise from the gut epithelium and remain *in situ* (Penttilä, 1968).

2) They arise from the gut epithelium and move out (Masson, 1923; his 'neuroentoderm').

3) They arise outside the epithelium and move in (Danisch, 1924; his neuro-argentaffin relationships).

We consider that the present evidence supports the third possibility but falls short of providing the necessary proofs for refutation of the first two propositions. Absolute proof for and origin of gut and pancreatic endocrine cells from neural ectoderm is unlikely to be obtained by the grafting techniques of conventional experimental embryology. Nor can these techniques be expected to provide acceptable evidence of a contrary state of affairs. For the time being it is necessary to rely on circumstantial evidence derived from studies in a number of different disciplines.

Quantitative studies of the development of endocrine cells can usefully be extended to the human embryo where they may be expected to provide valuable information concerning the physiological role of the various hormones in the period before and after the birth of the infant.

Acknowledgements

This work was carried out with the support of grants from the Medical Research Council, the Volkswagenwerk Stiftung and the Cancer Research Campaign.

References

Bloom, S R et al (1975) *Gut, 16,* 821
Carvalheira, A F et al (1968) *Histochemie, 14,* 33
Coons, A H et al (1955) *Journal of Experimental Medicine, 102,* 69
Cordier, E (1929) *Archives de Biologie, 36,* 427
Creutzfeldt, W et al (1970) In *Origin, Chemistry, Physiology and Pathophysiology of the Gastrointestinal Hormones.* Proceedings of International Symposium, Wiesbaden, 1969. Schattauer, Stuttgart and New York. Page 95.

Danisch, F (1924) *Beitraege zur Pathologischen Anatomie und Allgemeinen Pathologie,* 72, 687

Eränkö, O (1955) *Acta Endocrinologica,* 18, 174

Eränkö, O (1967) *Journal of the Royal Microscopical Society,* 87, 259

Esterhuizen, A C (1959) *South African Medical Journal,* 33, 197

Falck, B and Torp, A (1961) *Medicina Experimentalis (Basel),* 5, 429

Ferreira, D (1957) *Journal of Ultrastructure Research,* 1, 14

Feyrter, F (1938) *Über diffuse endokrine epitheliale Organe.* Barth, Leipzig.

Feyrter, F (1953) *Über die peripheren endokrinen (parakrinen) Drusen des Menschen.* 2nd ed. Wilhelm Maudrich, Vienna

Forssman, W G (1970) In *Origin, Chemistry, Physiology and Pathophysiology of the Gastrointestinal Hormones.* Proceedings of International Symposium, Wiesbaden, 1969. Schattauer, Stuttgart and New York. Page 31.

Forssman, W G et al (1969) *Journal of Cell Biology,* 40, 692

Frye, B E (1958) *Journal of Morphology,* 101, 325

Fujita, T (1973) *Gastro-entero-pancreatic endocrine system. A cell-biological approach.* (Ed.) T Fujita. Igaku Shoin Ltd, Tokyo, Japan

Golosow, N and Grobstein, C (1962) *Developmental Biology,* 4, 242

Grillo, T A I (1964) *Journal of Endocrinology,* 31, 67

Grüneburg, H (1943) *Journal of Heredity,* 34, 89

Hard, W L (1944) *American Journal of Anatomy,* 75, 369

Hellman, B (1965/66) *Biology of the Neonate,* 9, 263

Kobayashi, S et al (1970) *Archivum Histologicum Japonicum,* 31, 477

Kull, H (1913) *Archiv fur Mikrobiologie,* 81, 185

Kull, H (1925) *Zeitschrift fur Mikroskopisch-Anatomische Forschung,* 2, 163

Laguesse, E (1869) *Journal of Anatomy and Physiology,* 32, 209

Larsson, L I et al (1975) *Gastroenterology,* 68, 1152

Le Douarin, N (1969) *Bulletin Biologique de la France et de la Belgique,* 103, 435

Le Douarin, N and Le Lievre, C (1971) *Comptes Rendus de l'Association des Anatomistes,* 152, 558

Le Douarin, N et al (1972) *Comptes Rendus Hebdomadaires des Séances de l'Acadamie des Sciences (Paris),* 275, 583

Masson, P (1914) *La glande endocrine de l'intestine chez l'homme.*

Masson, P (1923) *Annales d'Anatomie Pathologique,* 1, 3

McAlpine, R J (1951) *Anatomical Record,* 109, 189 ·

Monesi, V (1960) *Acta Anatomica,* 41, 97

Munger, B L (1958) *American Journal of Anatomy,* 103, 275

Orci, L et al (1968) *Diabetologia,* 4, 56

Osaka, M et al (1971) *Archivum Histologicum Japonicum,* 33, 247

Parat, M (1924a) *Comptes Rendus des Séances de la Société de Biologie et de ses Filiales,* 90, 1023

Parat, M (1924b) *Comptes Rendus de l'Association des Anatomistes,* 19, 232

Pearse, A G E (1966a) *Nature (London),* 211, 598

Pearse, A G E (1966b) *Veterinary Record,* 79, 587

Pearse, A G E (1968) *Proceedings of the Royal Society of London (Biology),* 170, 71

Pearse, A G E (1969) *Journal of Histochemistry and Cytochemistry,* 17, 303

Pearse, A G E and Carvalheira, A F (1967) *Nature (London),* 214, 929

Pearse, A G E and Polak, J M (1971a) *Histochemie,* 27, 96

Pearse, A G E and Polak, J M (1971b) *Gut,* 12, 783

Pearse, A G E and Polak J M (1975) *Histochemical Journal,* 7, 179

Pearse, A G E et al (1974) *Histochemical Journal,* 6, 347

Pearse, A G E et al (1973a) *Diabetologia,* 9, 120

Pearse, A G E et al (1973b) *Histochemie,* 34, 191

Pearse, A G E and Takor, T (1976) *Journal of Clinical Endocrinology* (In press)

Penttilä, A (1968) *Annales Medicinae Experimentalis et Biologiae Fenniae,* 46, 457

Perrier, H (1970) *Diabetologia,* 6, 605

Pictet, R et al (1968) *Journal of Cell Biology,* 39, 105a (Abstract)

Pictet, R et al (1971) *Diabetes,* 20, suppl.I, 326

Polak, J M et al (1971a) *Gut, 12,* 311
Polak, J M et al (1971b) *Gut, 12,* 605
Polak, J M et al (1973) *Gut, 14,* 284
Polak, J M et al (1974a) *Gut, 15,* 720
Polak, J M et al (1974b) *Histochemistry, 40,* 209
Polak, J M et al (1971c) *General and Comparative Endocrinology, 16,* 132
Polak, J M et al (1972) *Gut, 13,* 501
Sasagawa, T et al (1970) *Archivum Histologicum Japonicum, 32,* 275
Sharples, W (1945) *Anatomical Record, 91,* 107
Simard, L D and van Campenhout, E (1932) *Anatomical Record, 53,* 141
Solcia, E et al (1969) *Histochemie, 20,* 116
Solcia, E et al (1970) In *Origin, Chemistry, Physiology and Pathophysiology of the Gastro-
intestinal Hormones.* Proceedings of International Symposium, Wiesbaden, 1969.
Schattauer, Stuttgart and New York.
Spooner, B S et al (1970) *Journal of Cell Biology, 47,* 245
Wessells, N K and Rutter, W J (1969) *Scientific American, 220,* 36

Discussion

PROFESSOR WILLIAMS One of the things that intrigues me most is the neural crest origin of the gut endocrine cells. I thought you hedged slightly by saying that it is proven for some, but not proven for other types. It is proven for C cells, I will accept that. Could you tell us what other cells it is proven for and could you comment on the work of Dr Ann Andrew who looked at the gut from the aganglionic segment in Hirschsprung's disease and said that argentaffin cells occurred there normally and therefore she thought they were not of neural origin?

POLAK Perhaps she is right. It has been proven in 'C' cells and the carotid body cells and the adrenal medullary cells but not in the gut. All we have seen are cells which have their characteristics and they occur in early embryos. We see them in the gastrointestinal tract, but there is a big gap and we do not see them migrating and reaching the gut.

WILLIAMS But does it enter the mucosa?

POLAK Well, we don't see them doing so. Our work is static, we see them in stages, the only way it could be proven is by the work of Le Douarin, in France, where they work mainly in birds and they have a biological marker; the quail cells have a special characteristic in their nuclei. They implant them into the chick and then the cells locate in the final organs. This would be the final proof but she is unable yet to find gut cells with quail characteristics.

42

DR MARGOT SHINER I am interested. You say for instance that in the mouse embryo you can stain the clear cells and yet they have very few granules. When you see the fluorescent stains with antiserum to particular cells, in morphological terms, what exactly do you stain, is it the granules or is it the cytoplasm?

POLAK There is no complete certainty about what we stain. There is quite strong evidence that we stain the granules and our work in mice would support that because when the granules are very immature, the staining reactions are very feeble, and we do not get any immuno-cytochemistry, whereas from the stage of 14 days onwards the granules become mature and immunofluorescence is possible. There is recent work from France in G cells suggesting that you can stain granular and nongranular forms but in our experience we have no evidence other than saying it is probably the granules that are stained.

Development of Immunological Mechanisms in the Gut

MARGOT SHINER

The gastrointestinal tract is well equipped to generate immunological reactions. It is undisputable that the gut should be regarded as a central lymphoid tissue. However, it is greatly disputed whether it bears any resemblance to the Bursa of Fabricius of birds (Figure 1) which controls the immunoglobulin-secreting cells that effect humoral immunity. In mammals these cells may develop in the fetal liver, possibly the spleen, and the aggregations of lymphoid follicles and germinal centres known as Peyer's patches.

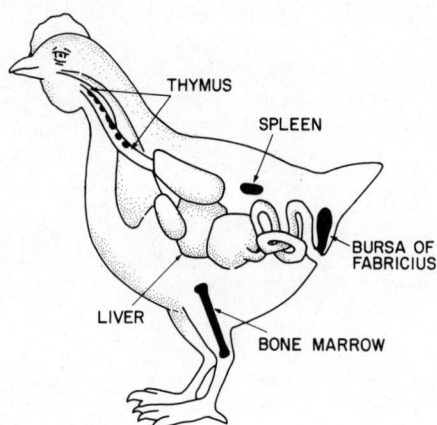

Figure 1. Bursa of Fabricius.

Lymphoid cells obtained from different sources have characteristic patterns of migration. Gowans and Knight (1964) found that tritium-labelled small lymphocytes obtained from the thoracic duct of rats 'homed' to the lymph nodes, spleen and Peyer's patches of syngeneic recipients, whereas the large lymphocytes migrated mostly to the stroma of the intestinal villi where they assumed the appearances of plasma cells. Griscelli and his co-workers (1969) observed that intravenously-injected large lymphoid cells from mesenteric, but not peripheral lymph nodes, travelled preferentially to the intestine.

44

Peyer's Patches

This lympho-epithelial tissue is concentrated in the lamina propria of the mucosa and in the submucosa of the ileum but extends upwards into the jejunum. The patches are well developed in man by about the 5th month of fetal life. They increase in size and in number later in gestation and continue this growth pattern for at least 10 years after birth. They involute in old age. The exact relationship of the Peyer's patches to the non-aggregated lymphoid tissue in the normal gut is not known but it is of interest to note that in the Bruton type of hypogamma-globulinaemia, characterised by a defect in the efferent limb of humoral (B-cell dependent) immunity, there is a lack of lymphoid tissue which affects, amongst other organs, the appendix. In germ-free animals the germinal centres of Peyer's patches as well as plasma cells are deficient and diminished, both becoming more conspicuous after antigenic exposure. This however is still no direct proof that the aggregated lymphoid tissue (Peyer's patches) is the precursor of the non-aggregated lymphocytes and plasma cells which populate the normal human gut. Isolated lymph nodules in the jejunal mucosa are a moderately frequent finding in young children and it may be of interest that few if any immunoctyes (immunoglobulin containing plasma cells) are found within them.

The Appendix

Another gut-associated lympho-epithelial tissue suspected of being the equivalent of the avian bursa of Fabricius is the appendix. Bockman and Cooper (1975) studied the appendices of fetuses, infants and young children. A definite develop-mental relationship between lymphoid follicles and the specialisation of the covering epithelium was shown, similar to that described in the Peyer's patches in the human and the bursa of Fabricius in the chickens. They suggested that this follicle-associated epithelium provides the necessary antigenic pathways which may stimulate clonal proliferation of B-lymphocytes in the underlying lymph follicles and seed them to other parts of the intestinal tract.

Local Antibody Synthesis

A number of studies have implied that by the 7th month of gestation the human fetus has developed a competent immune system. The initiation of immuno-globulin synthesis in the human newborn follows and is accelerated by exposure to antigens in the gut lumen. These antigens include a wide variety of chemical haptens, microbes, plant substances and dietary proteins. Antibodies to bovine serum albumin are formed early in neonatal life and their presence in the serum of these infants suggests that either whole protein molecules or at least their anti-genic fractions can be absorbed intact. Circulating antibodies to cow's milk can be demonstrated even in premature infants soon after birth and should be regarded as physiological.

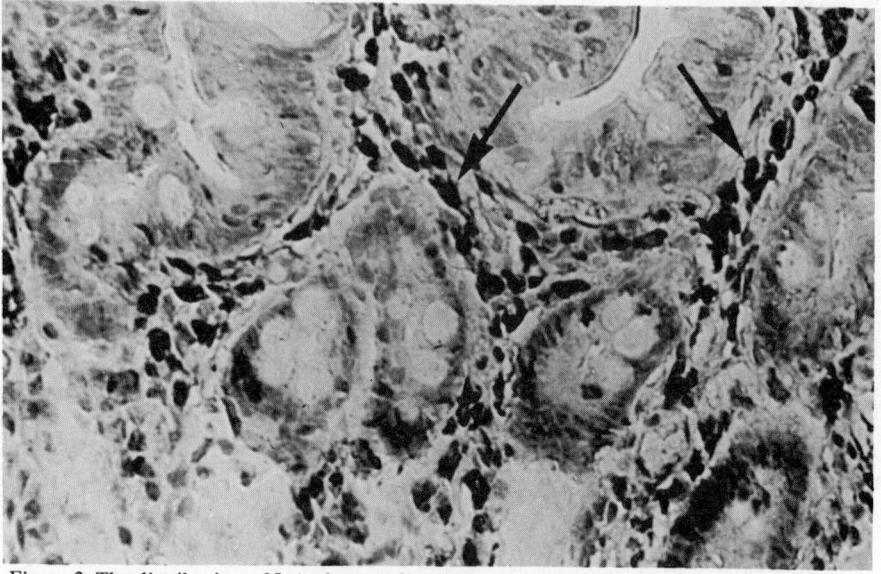

Figure 2. The distribution of IgA plasma cells within the normal jejunal mucosa. The brown staining (black in the photograph) of the IgA plasma cells is achieved by an immuno-histochemical technique, using horseradish peroxidase conjugated antisera to IgA on paraffin embedded sections. The villous and crypt epithelium has been counterstained blue (here dark grey). (× 28 approx.)

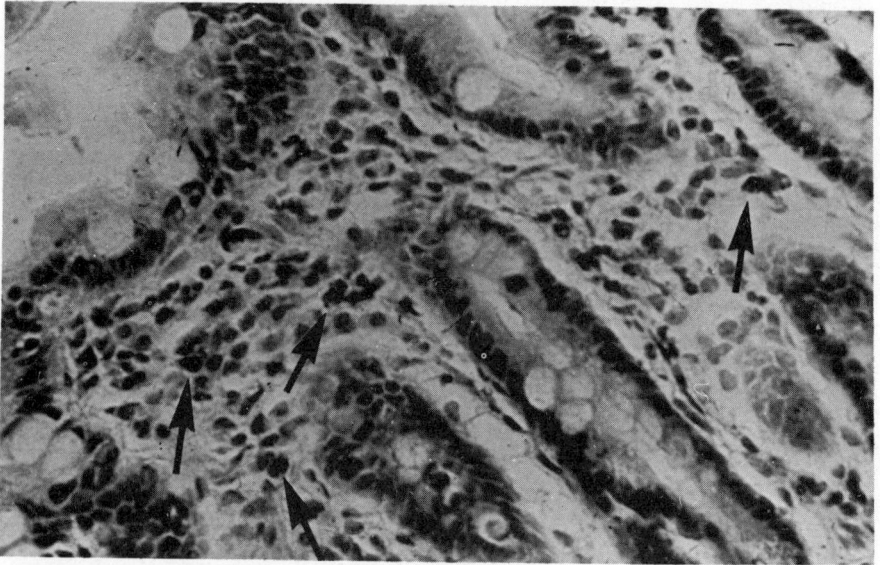

Figure 3. The distribution of IgM plasma cells. Same technique as Figure 2. (× 28 approx).

46

The Development of Specific Gut Immunoglobulins

IgA The intestine of the human fetus does not contain plasma cells producing this specific immunoglobulin. However, they appear in the newborn intestinal tract even before serum IgA is detectable. IgA plasma cells are the most numerous in the intestinal mucosa and the IgA is of the 7S variety. It is secreted into the lumen, after combining with secretory component, as a dimer of 11S IgA. The secretory component (Tomasi, 1968) is produced by the epithelium and is a glycoprotein. 11S IgA is certainly anti-viral but only possibly anti-bacterial. IgA in the intestinal mucosa and the external secretions has long been thought of as the most important immunoglobulin class of the gut and important protective functions are attributed to it. Certainly, the maternal colostrum and breast milk contain large amounts of 11S IgA which is said to be a source of protection to the infant, at least in the first 6 months of life. Although serum IgA is very low during the first 12 months (26–95 mg%) our work with immunofluorescence of the jejunal mucosa has shown surprisingly large numbers of IgA plasma cells, roughly equalling those of adults.

IgM This is the largest and also the most primitive immunoglobulin class. In the human gut IgM plasma cells are probably produced in the 3rd trimester before birth. The number of mucosal IgM plasma cells in relation to IgA cells is in the region of 20:7 and they are 7 times more numerous than IgG plasma cells.

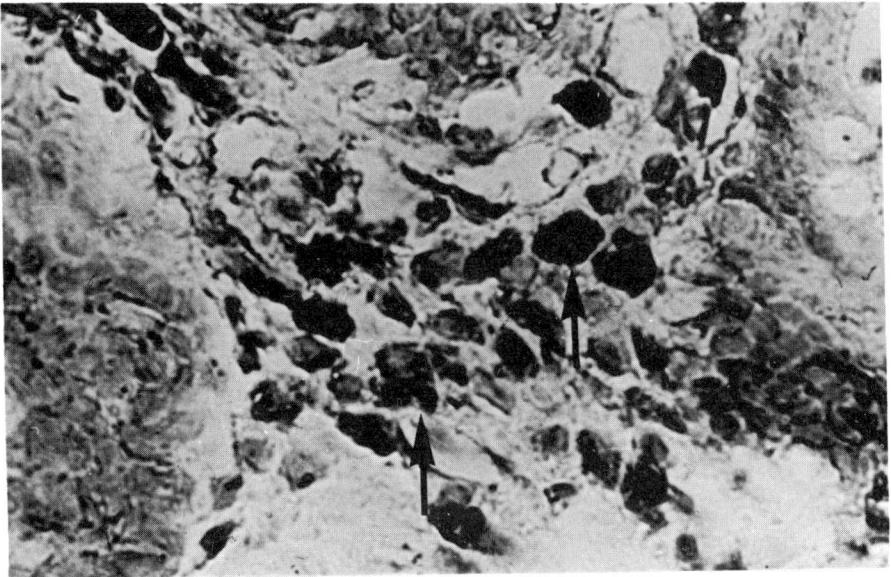

Figure 4. IgA staining plasma cells at higher magnification. (× 60 approx.)

47

Their exact function is ill-understood but in immune deficiency states they are often the last of the functioning plasma cells to remain in the gut. This applies particularly to selective IgA deficiency. IgM is also found in the external secretions and may combine with secretory component similarly to IgA.

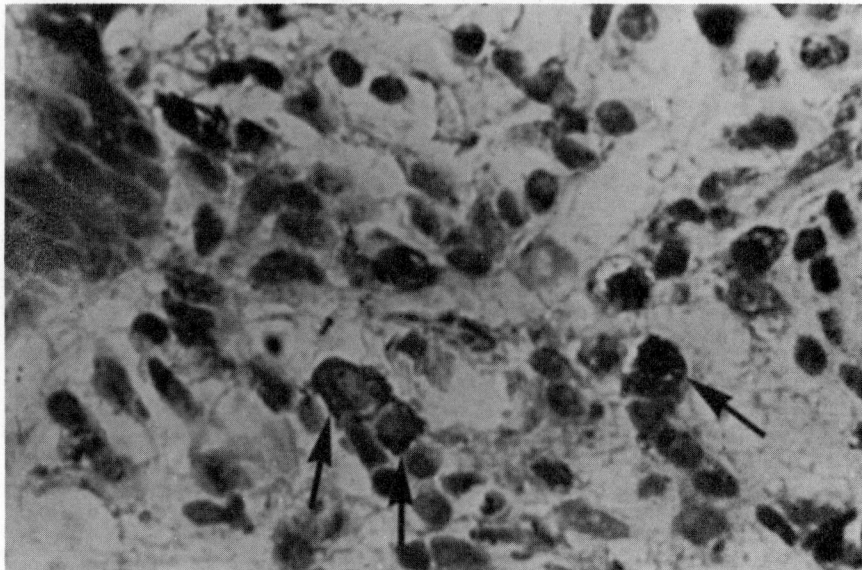

Figure 5. IgM staining plasma cells at higher magnification. These are far fewer than IgA plasma cells. Note the cytoplasm of the plasma cells staining brown (black in the photograph) and the nuclei staining blue (here dark grey). (X 60 approx.)

IgG In man IgG is the only immunoglobulin capable of crossing the placental barrier. This gives the fetus passive immunity to many environmental organisms though poor protection against Gram-negative bacteria. At least in animals it was shown that IgG can be selectively transported across the upper third of the small intestine. IgG plasma cells are few in the human intestinal mucosa and most of the IgG reaches the tissue via the blood. In common with IgM, it can bind complement, thus forming cytotoxic complexes within the mucosa.

IgE Whereas IgM, IgG and IgA probably arise from a common stem cell, IgE as well as IgD may arise from a separate cell line. At birth serum IgE levels are unmeasureable. By contrast we have found large numbers of IgE plasma cells in the jejunal mucosa of 3-month-old infants. The number of IgE plasma cells is similar to IgM plasma cells, a finding confirmed by others investigating the distribution of these cells throughout the gut. IgE-producing plasma cells appear to be

48

concentrated in mucosal tissues exposed to allergens, such as the nose, respiratory system, stomach, small intestine and rectum, and therefore have a similar distribution to IgA plasma cells. Serum IgA deficiency is said to have a high frequency in children with atopic disease (Taylor et al, 1973), although we have not been able to substantiate this by immunofluorescence of the jejunal mucosa in the case of milk allergy.

IgD   Little is known about the distribution and function of this immunoglobulin. Plasma cells containing IgD immunoglobulin have been demonstrated in the gut but they are very few in number.

A lymphoid cell type whose function has yet to be determined is the *theliolymphocyte* (Fichtelius, 1968). This cell is found between the epithelial cells of villi and crypts and resembles an immature lymphocyte characterised by an abundance of cytoplasm containing numerous ribosomes but little endoplasmic reticulum. They appear to move from the lamina propria, since they can be observed to penetrate the basal laminae of the epithelial cells, into the interepithelial spaces, but they are hardly ever observed in the gut lumen overlying the epithelium. It is therefore assumed that the theliolymphocytes shuttle to and fro, picking up antigenic material as they do so. Certain diseases, like untreated coeliac disease, show a great and measurable increase in theliolymphocytes.

Relationships Between Immunological Systems

The immune function of the gut appears to be largely independent of the immune system of the whole body. Serum immunoglobulins do not reflect increases or decreases of gut immunoglobulin production except in hypo- or agammaglobulinaemic states.

The role of cell mediated immunity (a function of thymus-derived or T-cell immunity) in relation to humoral or B-cell derived immunity within the gut is not clear. It is widely assumed that T-cells have to interact with B-cells in order for the latter to function and this would also apply to the gut. Even if the B-lymphocytes are derived from Peyer's patches (the equivalent of the Bursa of Fabricius), the origin of the T-cells in the gut is unknown. Some evidence has been produced that the theliolymphocytes might represent the T-cell line, picking up antigenic material on its surface from external secretions and relating it back to the B-lymphocyte which is thus stimulated to produce antibody. The gut also has numerous macrophages whose function is an important link in the interaction of local T- and B-cells.

49

References

Bockman, D E and Cooper, M (1975) *Gastroenterology, 68,* 1160
Fichtelius, K E (1968) *Experimental Cell Research, 49,* 87
Gowans, J L and Knight, E J (1964) *Proceedings of the Royal Society (Biol), 159,* 257
Griscelli, C, Vassalli, P and McCluskey, R T (1969) *Journal of Experimental Medicine, 130,* 1427
Tomasi, T B Jr (1968) *New England Journal of Medicine, 279,* 1327
Taylor, B, Norman, A P, Orgel, H A, Turner, M W, Stokes, C R and Soothill, J R (1973) *Lancet, ii,* 111

Discussion

CHAIRMAN   At what stage is it thought that IgA cells become competent in embryonic life?

SHINER   It is not known, but apparently the plasma cells do not produce IgA until after birth.

CHAIRMAN   Do you find IgA in the faeces of a normal infant?

SHINER   Yes, you should have IgA in faeces.

CHAIRMAN   Do you think it could come from the breast milk, if the child is breast fed?

SHINER   It comes from both sources. Most of the IgA is said to come from the colostrum and from breast milk in small infants, but I find it very surprising that such large numbers of IgA-producing or IgA-staining plasma cells are found in a very young child. The earliest we have found are from two months onwards and the numbers are really considerable. This is not reflected in the serum of these children.

Development of Liver Function

A P MOWAT

The liver plays an important role in the metabolic homeostasis of the mammalian organism. The differentiation and biochemical maturation of the liver is thus of considerable importance in determining growth, development and functioning of other tissues, and understanding of its functional maturation explains the specific effects of temporary hepatic inefficiency in the newborn period.

The liver is formed at an early stage in embryonic life from an invagination of the foregut into the septum transversum. By late gestation morphological characteristics of liver cells are well developed but most enzymes concerned with the homeostatic functions of the liver are of negligible activity since many of these functions of the liver are at this time performed by the placenta and maternal tissues. Changes in function in the perinatal period are mediated by intra- and extrahepatic vascular changes together with extensively studied but only partially understood, changes in enzymatic activity. Many of the enzymatic studies have had to be performed in vitro from tissues of experimental animals and often using substrates which are not the natural substrates for the enzyme, so that extrapolation of experimental findings to the intact human is hazardous. A further technical problem is that comparisons between fetal and adult liver are often based on activities expressed in grams of weight of liver, although it is known that the liver in the newborn contains a relatively large amount of water, substantial amounts of haemopoetic tissue and considerably less protein than the adult.

There would appear to be little doubt, however, that there is a transient period following birth when homeostasis may be unstable, perhaps because of low enzymatic activity, and we as paediatricians must be very careful not to aggravate this by the care offered to newborn infants. It is perhaps worth recalling that in the light-for-dates infant, the liver mass is disproportionately reduced compared with body and brain weight; they may thus have an additional handicap.

We have much to learn of the factors which control hepatic activity. An increase in enzymatic activity may arise from increased synthesis or decreased degradation. Synthesis can certainly be influenced by the amount of substrate present, but exactly how this acts is not clear. Metabolic effects not directly related to the metabolic pathway in which the enzyme plays a role, may also be important. For example, if we consider the enzyme tyrosine alpha-ketoglutarate transaminase, enzymatic activity of this enzyme may be increased by hypoglycaemia which induces glucagon release and production of cyclic AMP which in its turn increases enzymatic activity. Corticosteroids and adrenaline have a similar effect although not necessarily mediated through cyclic AMP but these, however, only act post-natally (Adams, 1971). In most circumstances, it is not known whether such effects are due to the increased synthesis or decreased degradation of the enzyme or merely activation of already present enzymatic protein. A striking example of in vivo activation of enzymatic activity is to be found by studying the activity of glucuronyl transferase in the developing chick. Prior to hatching, this enzyme is present in appreciable concentration but the moment the chick bursts into the air sac within the shell or bursts from the shell, enzymatic activity increased three-fold to levels greater than in the adult. It subsequently falls to somewhat lower levels at the fourth day, and then rises thereafter (Dutton, 1963).

In vitro activation of glucuronyl transferase is illustrated in Table I. This shows that when enzymatic activity is determined in the presence of diethylnitrosamine the apparent activity is increased in all instances by a factor of < 3. This is particularly striking when liver tissue from the Gunn rat is used since this animal has a congenital unconjugated hyperbilirubinaemia, like the human with Crigler-Najjar Syndrome, usually attributed to deficiency of UDP glucuronyl transferase. The Table also illustrates the low activity of the enzyme found in hypophysectomised and thyroidectomised rats.

TABLE I. Activation of o-aminophenol glucuronide formation in vitro by diethylnitrosamine
(Nmoles/mg protein/20 min)

Tissue source	Diethyl Nitrosamine	
	Absent	Present
Normal rat	27	58
Hypophysectomised	3.0	38
Thyroidectomised	4·0	39
Gunn Rat	3·0	83

From the data of Mowat, A P and Arias, I M. *Biochemica and Biophysica, Acta, 1970, 212,* 175.

Detoxication Systems

The systems responsible for detoxication are present in low activities in newborn liver (Lathe, 1974). Two main mechanisms are involved, oxidative detoxication requiring NADP and oxygenation, and conjugation with glucuronic acid, sulphates, acetylates or glutathione. Both processes convert toxic substances, drugs and hormones into less active derivatives which are excreted in the bowel or urine. There is little doubt that both processes are handicapped in the human newborn.

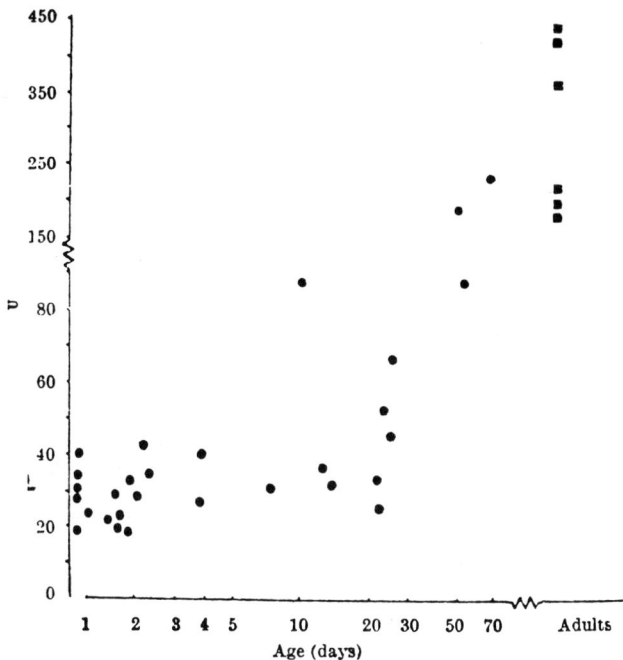

Figure 1. Glucuronyl transferase activity expressed as a percentage of the adult value (100%) from G H Lathe (1974) in *Scientific Foundations of Paediatrics*, p. 108

If we were to ask paediatricians for an example, they would no doubt quote transient neonatal hyperbilirubinaemia due to low UDP glucuronyl transferase activity, having in mind some chart, such as that shown in Figure 1 which shows low UDP glucuronyl transferase activity in the newborn period rising gradually soon after birth, a pattern of development mirroring neonatal physiological jaundice, overlooking that the species tested had no physiologic jaundice. The only study of this enzyme activity done in human biopsy material, however, shows a totally different time course of development, not reaching adult levels until about the 70th day. In this study, however, the substrate was not bilirubin (Figure 2). This is a striking illustration of how species and substrate may influence the results of laboratory investigations. This is not to say that there is no impaired excretion of bilirubin and other aglycones in the human newborn. Many endogenous and exogenous substances do not undergo glucuronide conjugation as rapidly in the newborn as later in life. Alternate explanations such as ineffective hepatic perfusion, inefficient hepatic uptake of bilirubin and lack of an ion-binding transport protein, such as Ligandin, in the hepatic cytoplasm as well as increased enteric reabsorption of the aglycones, must be considered as well as an inefficient glucuronide formation.

53

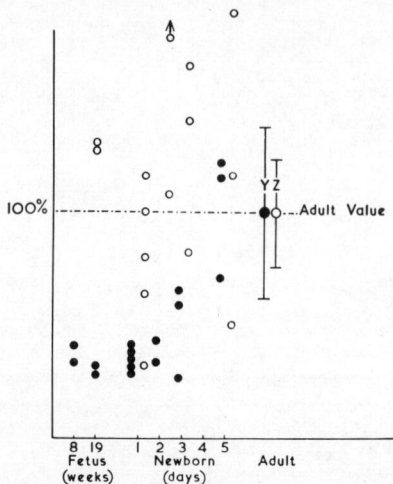

Figure 2. UDP glucuronyl transferase activity determined in percutaneous liver biopsies in infants, using methyl-umpelliferone, from the data of D'Toro, R, Lupi, L, and Ansanelli, V (1968) *Nature* (London), *219*, 265

Protein Synthesis

Protein synthesis is very active in the fetal liver. Some of this, however, may represent haemopoietic activity rather than hepatocyte function. The serum protein alpha-fetoprotein is of some interest. It first appears in the serum at the 6-week embryo stage rising to a peak concentration of 300 mg/100 ml at 13 weeks' gestation and then declines linearly to around 7 mg/100 ml in the cord serum at term. The concentration thereafter falls rapidly to levels of between 100 and 1700 ng/100 ml.

In contrast albumin synthesis starts at approximately 3–4 months gestation and gradually increases, but low levels are commonly found in prematurely born infants. The concentration of specific plasma proteins involved in, for example, coagulation, is frequently low around the time of delivery, and more strikingly that of the protein caerulo-plasmin remains very low in the first two to three months of life, indicating clearly that there is no uniformity in the development of hepatic protein synthesis.

Although all amino acids except cystine, are in higher concentration in fetal blood than in the adult, the enzymes involved in the metabolism or degradation of amino acids are of low activity in fetal liver (Räitha, 1974). For example, methionine is converted through homocysteine to cystathionine then through the action of the enzyme cystathionase to cysteine, which in its turn may be metabolised to cystine, as well as taurine, and sulphate. However, cystathionase activity develops post-natally in the human liver and, as a result, we see in healthy premature infants high cystathioninurea, and in infants who are given

54

a high protein diet, high methionine levels are also found. Conversely, cysteine may be an essential amino acid for premature infants.

If we now consider phenylalanine degradation to acetyl-coenzyme A, the first step in its conversion to tyrosine takes place in the presence of the enzyme phenylalanine 4-hydroxylase. The elevated phenylalanine levels in prematures has been attributed to deficiency of this enzyme. However, much conflicting data exists about the frequency of this. Some have reported good tolerance of phenylalanine load with high urinary tyrosine excretion, but others have reported decreased tolerance. It is found, however, that if premature infants are given 100 mg of ascorbic acid per day, both phenylalanine and tyrosine concentrations fall to normal indicating that it is not the lack of the enzyme but of a vital co-factor which causes the inefficient amino acid metabolism. Clearly, if we are to feed our premature infants a diet high in protein and low in ascorbic acid, this will aggravate the problem. Usually by the time the infant is one week of age a normal response to phenylalanine loading may be seen, but this is not so in all cases.

While most reports suggest that this is a benign lesion, a follow-up study at the age of 7 or 8 years of age in children who had transitory tyrosinaemia correlated this with abnormalities of visual perception and caused the authors to speculate that high protein feeding of premature infants could be the cause of some instances of minimal brain damage (Menkes et al, 1972).

Another area of concern to paediatricians is the hepatic role in carbohydrate metabolism in the newborn period. Large amounts of glycogen appear in the liver towards the end of gestation and are mobilised very rapidly after birth in all mammalian species (Adams, 1971). This rapid hepatic synthesis of glycogen appears to be under the control of the pituitary-adrenal axis. There seems to be some species variation in the main sources of glycogen but generally, glucose, fructose, galactose, and pyruvates may be incorporated. There are probably important species differences in the capacity for glyconeogenesis by the fetal liver. The factors that influence these in utero changes in metabolism are not known. Post-natally, changes in the involved enzymes can be determined. These can generally be related to the diet taken at the time. Following birth, there is activation of alpha-glucan phosphorylase induced by the hormones adrenaline or glucagon. A sharp increase in activity is presumably related to the mobilisation of liver glycogen at this time. The tendency of newborn animals to hypoglycaemia cannot, however, be attributed to low activity of any of the known enzymes of glycogen breakdown, but it is possible that the post-natal development of glyconeogenesis is not sufficiently rapid to immediately replenish liver glycogen stores.

In my review of the development of hepatic function, I have concentrated on the perinatal period, since it is at this stage that the organism is adapting to an independent existence without the support of maternal and placental metabolism. The factors involved in the control of the increased enzymatic activity after birth are still largely a matter for speculation. The most obvious mechanism is the accumulation of substrate which can no longer be removed by the placenta and increased activity mediated by adrenal and pancreatic endocrine changes associated with the stress of birth.

There are possibly important teleological reasons for the differences in liver function in the neonate compared with the adult. If we try to modify one aspect of hepatic function, e.g. by giving phenobarbitone to prevent hyperbilirubinaemia, we may inadvertently adversely affect other aspects of metabolism. Drugs given during pregnancy, delivery and post-natally, vascular effects of respiratory distress syndrome or its ventilatory treatment as well as feeding regimens are examples of factors influencing hepatic function. Indeed, when we modify the intrauterine, perinatal or post-natal environment in any way adverse effects on liver function may occur.

References

Adams, P (1971) Control of glucose metabolism in the Human Fetus and Newborn Infant. *Advances in Metabolic Disorders, 5,* (Ed) Levine & Luft. Academic Press, New York. Page 183

Dutton, G J (1973) Glucuronide formation. *Annals of New York Acad. Sciences, III,* 259

Boesman, M (1966) Serum Alphafetoprotein, albumin and globulin synthesis in the human conceptus. *Journal of Clinical Investigation, 45,* 126

Lathe, G H (1974) Neonatal Jaundice; Bile pigment metabolism in the fetus and newborn infant. *Scientific Foundation of Paediatrics,* (Ed) J A Davis & J J Dobbing. Heinemann, London. Page 105

Menkes, J H, Welcher, D W et al (1972) Relationship of Elevated blood tyrosine to the ultimate intellectual performance of premature infants. *Paediatrics, 49,* 212

Myant, N B (1971) Developmental aspects of lipid metabolism. *The Biochemistry of Development,* (Ed) P F Benson. Heinemann, London. Page 96

Räitha, N C R (1974) Perinatal Metabolism of some enzymes of amino acid metabolism in the liver. *Scientific Foundation of Paediatrics,* (Ed) J A Davis & J Dobbing. Heinemann, London

Discussion

DR R G WILSON   I was a little confused when you were talking about the liver in the small-for-dates baby. You said the liver was smaller, which everyone will accept, and you implied that there was a limited reserve of liver function. Now is it small because there is less water, less nitrogen or less cells?

MOWAT   No, I did not mean to imply that I had any special knowledge of hepatic reserves in the small baby. I only wanted to make the point that the liver was small in small-for-dates babies. I do not know anything about the reserves.

DR A D GRIFFITHS   Is there any evidence that there are inhibitors of enzyme activity at birth and that the level of these inhibitors alters?

56

MOWAT   Well, I can only talk with confidence of glucuronyl transferase and say that there is no evidence of inhibitive activity at birth except for a few special instances in families of mothers carrying the serum hepatitis antigen and in some instances of the breast milk jaundice syndrome.

PROFESSOR GRAY   I wonder if I can ask you a question with regard to the transient tyrosinaemias? You said they were more likely to have CNS abnormalities when followed up. Could I ask you whether that work was based on comparison with controls of the same gestation and the same birth weight, because it is rather worrying in fact if they have got a liability to brain damage?

MOWAT   The children were seen at the age of eight years and had a comprehensive work-up using techniques which I have always used and which have been standardised on normal infants. They did not in this particular group compare with infants of low birth weight, nor in fact from the same unit, so there were other factors. This is a big problem in assessing minor CNS abnormalities: the further you get from the event the more difficult it is to make your first correlation.

QUESTION FROM AUDIENCE   How much does the fetus depend on its own liver function, and, also, when is intrahepatic circulation first established in normal life?

MOWAT   I find it very difficult to answer either of these questions. If a liver is badly damaged one does find infants born with cirrhosis and with oedema and low serum albumins and so on; and often it is rather like in an adult, very difficult to correlate function with morphological abnormalities. I do not know anything about when the intrahepatic circulation is switched on.

Panel Discussion
DEVELOPMENT OF THE GUT IN THE FETUS AND YOUNG CHILD

PROFESSOR WILLIAMS We have been discussing this morning the development of hormones, enzymes and antibodies. There are a considerable number of congenital syndromes that affect hormones, enzymes and antibodies in the gut and in the liver, and I wonder whether any of the experts who have been talking to us this morning know whether a defect in one of these mechanisms affects a defect in the other. For example, in the pancreas where you have abnormal islets in rhesus incompatibility or diabetes, does anything happen to the development of the enzymes in the exocrine cells? Or in the gut where you have one of the many immunological syndromes, does anything happen to the rest of the gut? I wonder if I could start the discussion off with that very general question.

PROFESSOR HADORN As far as the pancreas is concerned it is very interesting that the exocrine and the endocrine pancreas seem to be extremely independent, even in a disease which affects the exocrine pancreas very early, like Shwachman-Diamond syndrome which is a syndrome in which the exocrine cells are at a very early stage destroyed by an unknown process. In this syndrome, the islets of Langerhans are completely normal and well preserved, and there is no evidence of any dysfunction of the hormone secretion. The other problem is whether there is any exocrine disease in diabetes. This is not known. There has been a suggestion that there are perhaps certain problems with gut function, but not deficiency of exocrine pancreatic function.

DR MOWAT I think one of the problems in trying to answer a hypothetical question like this is that most enzymes are shared by all cells. Although one sees a cell, a hepatocyte for example, doing a particular metabolic task, in the total organism you can often demonstrate the same metabolic abnormality, for example in fibroblasts.

WILLIAMS I was speaking partly in terms of development. Now if all the endocrine cells in the gut are of neural crest origin, are there different environmental influences in different parts of the gut that let them differentiate in different ways, so that the cells in one place are associated with particular hormone production?

58

DR JULIA POLAK I would quote the work of Nicole Le Douarin. She put the upper neural crest of the quail, the one which gives rise to 'C' cells and calcitonin, in the lower portion of the adrenal medulla of the chick. She wanted to know whether they could produce calcitonin, and found that if the 'C' cells were in the wrong environment, then they could not do so.

DR PRICE Dr Polak mentioned the hypothalamic relationship of gut hormones and I was wondering if she could enlarge on this?

POLAK I couldn't really give the evidence, but there are two types of hypothalamic hormones. I would like to refer especially to the growth hormone release inhibiting hormone or somatostatin, which has been extracted from the hypothalamus. Some somatostatin-like immunoreactivity can be found in the pancreas and in the gut, where this hormone has powerful local actions. There is no good evidence that it is indeed the same hormone with the same aminoacid sequence and it may not be absolutely identical.

WILLIAMS I think it is not a question of hypothalamic control. It is a question of hypothalamic hormones being found in the gut.

MR FREEMAN Dr Shiner, in the paediatric surgical literature there has been a statement made recently that in babies with necrotising enterocolitis, even a single feed with breast milk will protect them against infection or will certainly lower the morbidity considerably. Would you like to comment on that?

DR MARGOT SHINER I haven't read this paper, but did they say that they did any studies in the gut? Was there a low IgA?

FREEMAN Well, they claimed that the first feed of milk was essential to give the baby some IgA, and if you didn't do this, his resistance was very much lower and he could succumb to necrotising enterocolitis, whereas a baby fed on breast milk having the same stimulus would not.

SHINER This is the old question: how essential is breast milk? We have not adequately studied newborns and the relation between IgA production in the gut and symptomatology. I think a study which would be well worthwhile would be to find out what is going on in the gut of the newborn and during the first month of life. How much immunity can the infant muster on its own without the help of breast milk?

DR LITTLEWOOD Dr Shiner said that the development of cow's milk antibodies in a newborn infant was physiological. I wonder if this is really correct? Is it really physiological to develop cow's milk antibodies? I think it is a bit like saying that smoker's cough is physiological. On the other hand, do you accept all the very old work on the amazing protective effect of breast milk? You can see it quoted quite often, the enormous improvements in mortality and morbidity in the breast fed. Do you think that our refined methods of treating diarrhoea in the infant have somewhat blunted the edge of this advantage of breast milk?

SHINER I do not know whether cow's milk antibodies are physiological. I think that the fact that you have circulating antibodies to cow's milk, without any symptoms in about 50% of normal infants, suggests that it is a normal state of affairs. It could be that these circulating antibodies are present in all infants at one stage and that some lose it and others do not, but it is certainly compatible with health to have circulating antibodies.

DR McNEISH I would like to support Dr Shiner in this. I think it *is* physiological on the grounds of recent work by Walker and Isselbacher (1974) on macromolecular absorption. They showed that it is certainly normal for the neonate to absorb small quantities of macromolecules. It is probably also normal for the adult, certainly the adult small mammal, and possibly man as well, to absorb tiny quantities of macromolecules which are nutritionally completely irrelevant but which are certainly not immunologically irrelevant. It is physiological for the body to respond to an injection of protein by producing antibodies. The circumstances , the dosage and the timing of the injection may vary the antibodies, but nevertheless that is physiology, so I think that cow's milk antibodies are physiological.

DR WALKER-SMITH May I just comment on the merits of breast milk in gastroenteritis? There is a lot of recent work, and I think the best data is from Chile where a community was entirely breast fed and then bottle fed and they had figures of the incidence of gastroenteritis before and after abandonment of breast feeding. I also heard recently of some data from Iraq which showed that the benefits of breast milk are larger when the baby is exclusively breast fed, and that even a complementary feed does diminish the protection against gastroenteritis. Certainly in our experience in the Queen Elizabeth Hospital, London, delayed recovery from gastroenteritis is consistent in the bottle fed infants.

DR PROSSER I wonder if Professor Hadorn could expand on something he said earlier about lactase deficiency in certain racial groups?

HADORN A lot has been written about this, and the best article is probably the one written by Norman Kretchmer in 'Scientific American' (1972). The theory is that tribes in Africa who have raised cattle have a higher level of lactase, and can tolerate lactose, better than those who have not raised cattle. But there are many assumptions that you must make, you must assume that they have gone through a selection process and that during the evolution of these tribes a situation has occurred where they actually depended on the milk of these cows, so that the lactase-deficient subjects were under heavy selective pressure. It could also be the other way around, that they have raised cattle because they tolerated lactose.

DR LEWIS I would like to ask Professor Hadorn about the relationship between the concentration of sucrase and lactase in the newborn infant. Would he speculate as to what the advantage might be to the newborn infant to have the ratios reversed?

HADORN From the small data we have in man, we can say that sucrase activity develops a little earlier than lactase, so that for example, a premature baby of 1,500 grammes will have a low lactase level.

    What are the implications? Lifshitz says that one should not feed these prematures a lactose containing milk as this may cause acidosis and he has supported this by some good evidence, but this appears to be the only opinion on this subject and it is not absolutely clear. A high lactose load is not very well dealt with even by the normal newborn, who excretes a stool which is acid on breast milk, but he certainly does not get acidosis. Maybe this is a little more serious in prematures or low birth weight infants.

LEWIS You observed that the enzyme activity in the newborn undergoes a sudden boost at birth and you said that this is under hormonal influence. I was not clear whether you meant this was an internal hormone effect, or what?

HADORN We studied this in the chick. Just before hatching there is a tremendous increase in protein synthesis. The factor which stimulates protein synthesis in this way has not been identified, but it occurs just before hatching. In the rat, increased synthesis of lactase occurs shortly before birth. It is due to a true increase in enzyme synthesis, not to activation of a precursor. It is not due to a *new* synthesis: the enzyme is already there, but its production is very much accelerated at this time. I cannot answer the question whether the stimulus is maternal or fetal, but even if the fetus is removed earlier from the uterus, by caesarean section, it does occur at the right time. It is an intrinsic phenomenon of the fetus.

References

Kretchmer, N (1972) *Scientific American, 227,* 71
Walker, W W, Isselbacher, K J and Bloch, K J (1974) *American Journal of Clinical Nutrition, 27,* 1434

Infancy and its Problems

The Fate of a Feed

BRIAN A. WHARTON

Food is essential, always affecting the quality of life and sometimes its very continuation. Food is handled at first by the gastrointestinal tract but eventually by
all the other systems. Other chapters in this book are concerned with the role of
the gastrointestinal tract in the handling of food; this chapter describes how
nutrients from very variable diets may begin their action within the gut lumen,
interact with each other during and after absorption, and then either be shunted
out of the body by the kidney or be assimilated into the general composition of
the body. The chapter is concerned with that process which was described in
1779 as follows by Albrecht von Haller in his 'First Lines of Physiology':

> 'A gelatinous juice is conveyed from the aliments through the arteries to all
> parts of the body, and exudes into the cellular texture everywhere.'

Variation in Diet

There is considerable geographical variation in our diet. Variation is so great between the diet of ourselves, the Eskimo (who takes only 3% of his energy as carbohydrate) and people in Japan (who take only 10% of their energy as fat), that
it is difficult to understand how three animals taking such a different diet can,
nevertheless, be more or less similar.

Also there is tremendous variation in diet according to the ages of man. During
the first few months of life he eats one single food which is wholly liquid, while
towards the end of the first year of life he eats a whole variety of food, some
liquid, some solid. This pattern is followed only in certain countries however; in
many developing countries weaning often does not occur until the end of the first
year of life. The time of weaning has become earlier and earlier in this country;
in the post-war years most children were not weaned before the age of six months,
now the vast majority are weaned by three months. This earlier weaning may have
associated problems, e.g. it may lead to obesity, to the earlier development of
coeliac disease, and to osmolar problems (DHSS, 1974) while in a developing
country weaning may be followed by kwashiorkor. Children who meet problems
at weaning are, nevertheless, the minority. The net effect of weaning for the

64

majority of children is very much the same no matter when or how they are weaned, or in which part of the world they are living. Even before weaning, however, there is considerable variation in nutrient intake, much more variation than occurs in later years. The child who receives cows' milk, by far the majority in this country, takes in, compared to one receiving breast milk, three times as much protein, protein of different quality, fat which is very different qualitatively, substantially less lactose, and substantially more minerals. Yet, although we may be concerned that a proportion of babies receiving breast milk run into such problems as hypocalcaemia, hyperosmolality and so on, the overall effects of cows' milk for the vast majority are similar to those of breast milk.

There are then variations in the diet of man, some depending on geographical and cultural factors, others on the developing requirements of the growing organism. Clearly they must be very elastic mechanisms which are able to take such a varied diet and produce more or less the same sort of organism.

Physiological Role of Non-absorbed Nutrients

Dietary constituents may have a physiological effect before they are absorbed or even when they are not absorbed at all.

If there is a lot of lactose in the diet as there is for example in breast milk, then this easily overcomes the ability of the upper gastrointestinal tract to absorb it, and it passes down to the ileum where it enhances the absorption of calcium, strontium and magnesium (Mills et al, 1940; Gerstley et al, 1945; Greenwald et al, 1963). This mechanism is probably not quantitatively important because children receiving a lactose free diet do not develop calcium problems. However, this point of intestinal physiology has led to an interesting anthropological speculation; Caucasians following a mutation, maintained lactase in their gut throughout their life and so they could carry on drinking milk even after weaning; some of the lactose which they continued to eat passed down into the ileum and so helped them to absorb calcium; they were, therefore, more fit to migrate from the tropics because their enhanced calcium absorption helped to prevent rickets as they disappeared from the sun. Perhaps this speculation does not pay enough attention to vitamin D metabolism but it is, nevertheless, an interesting one.

Leaving aside speculation, however, unabsorbed lactose has other physiological functions in the newborn child. Lactose, if it is not absorbed, passes into the lower gut and following bacterial fermentation results in acidic gut contents. Because in breast milk the concentration of buffering substances, such as casein and phosphate, are low the gut contents remain acid and this leads to a predominant growth in the faeces of lactobacilli, i.e. non-pathogenic commensals (Bullen & Willis, 1971).

Cows' milk contains much less lactose so that little of it passes into the large intestine; furthermore, the higher casein and phosphate content of cows' milk buffers any acidic tendency so that the faeces of the baby receiving cows' milk are relatively more alkaline which promotes the growth of *E.coli* rather than lactobacilli. There are other substances which, acting prior to their digestion and absorption, contribute to the differences in faecal flora between babies receiving breast milk or cows' milk. One of these is a breast milk protein, lactoferrin, which has a bacteriostatic effect on *E.coli*. If the lactoferrin is already saturated with iron, then it loses that anti-bacterial effect (Bullen et al, 1972). Lactoferrin may act alone or more powerfully by synergism with antibody. Breast milk contains maternal antibodies and some of these are found in the faeces of children receiving the breast milk. These physiologically active substances have gone right the way through the gastrointestinal tract without being broken down, mainly because they are in the form of secretory IgA (Kenny et al, 1967). There is some evidence that the IgG and the IgM present in breast milk are not quite so easily broken down as had previously been thought, but mostly antibodies present in faeces are in the IgA class. A non-absorbed nutrient has enabled the baby to borrow some of its mother's previous immunological experience and so obtain some temporary passive protection.

Although these examples of non-absorbed, but physiologically active substances are chosen from the paediatric age group, and mainly from the newborn, the principles are applicable to adults as well. Perhaps the best example of a non-absorbed, but physiologically active, substance in adults would be fibre (Nutrition Society, 1973).

Interaction of Nutrients During and Following Absorption

Whether or not the nutrients have a physiological role in the gut they will eventually be either digested and absorbed, or will pass into the faeces.

Much of our knowledge of absorption is based on studies on individual nutrients given, not as part of food but as an isolated substance. The reasons for this are easy to understand and indeed our understanding of intestinal handling of say amino acids has been considerably advanced by studying them in isolation either in man following a load, or perhaps in an everted sac or a closed loop of small intestine. Nevertheless, these are all unphysiological situations — we take in nutrients by eating them as food, not as individual substances; we rarely have free amino acids in our diet and almost never eat protein without eating fat and carbohydrate too.

Some of the differences between eating a nutrient as part of a food or as an isolated substance are illustrated in Figure 1 which shows the changes in plasma glucose and valine following a drink of milk, compared to the changes following the same amount of casein and lactose given as individual substances. Following milk, the rise in the plasma of glucose was significantly less than following lactose alone and the rise in plasma valine was below that following an equivalent amount of casein. Table I shows some of the possible explanations for the interaction of nutrients in this particular example, but the same principles could be applied to all other foods.

66

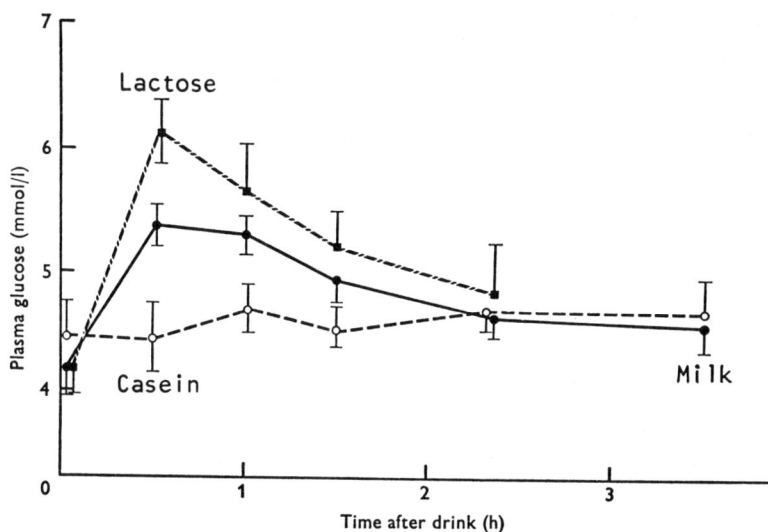

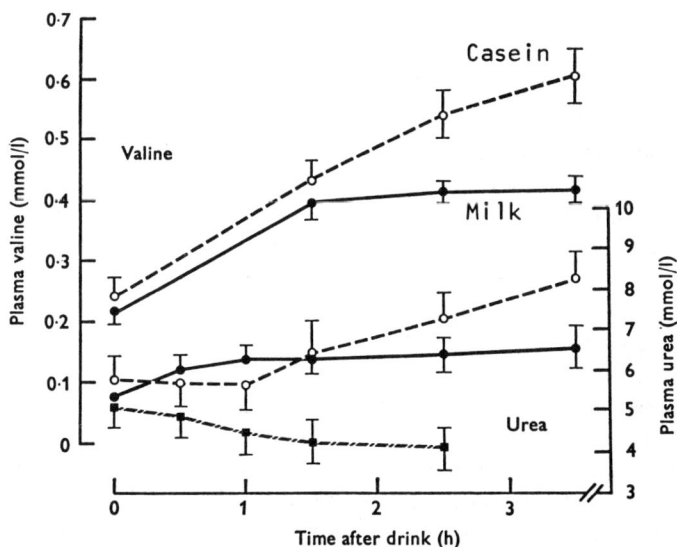

Figure 1. Plasma glucose, saline and urea (mean ± SE) in samples taken from children at various intervals, after drinks of milk casein or lactose. After milk (●–●) fifteen subjects; casein (0–0) eight subjects, and lactose (■–■) nine subjects, from Rossiter et al, 1974 – reproduced by kind permission editor *British Journal of Nutrition*

The initial inhibition of the active transport of amino acids and monosaccharides (Schultz & Curran, 1970; Cook, 1974) is a comparatively recent observation. The previous section of this chapter included an example of how happenings within the intestine had been built into evolutionary theory; in a similar way it has been

67

TABLE I. Interaction of Nutrients

Observations
(a) Plasma glucose rises less after milk than after lactose.
(b) Plasma essential amino acids rise less after milk than after casein.

Possible explanations
(a) *Gastric*
   Higher osmolar load of milk slows gastric emptying.
(b) *Intestinal*
   Mutual inhibition of active transport of amino acids and monosaccharides released from milk.
(c) *Metabolic and Hormonal*
   (i) Lack of carbohydrate in casein feed leads to decreased insulin production and reduced uptake of amino acids by muscle.
   (ii) Synergistic effect of amino acids, glucose, and galactose from milk on insulin production causes increased uptake of glucose and amino acids by cells.

Rossiter et al, 1974

suggested that in an environment where there is not much dietary protein then perhaps a mechanism which slowed down the rate of delivery of monosaccharides to the intestine could be an advantage because it would aid amino acid absorption; therefore, it could be an advantage for someone living on a low protein diet if they also had lactase deficiency, because the rate at which monosaccharides would be released into the enterocyte would be very much slower. This would be so long as the lactase deficiency was not so severe as to cause clinical diarrhoea.

The concentration in extracellular fluid of many nutrients is, of course, relatively independent of intestinal events and we have to be wary of 'wearing gastrointestinal blinkers', i.e. of interpreting changes in plasma levels of various nutrients purely in terms of gut handling. A well known example is that plasma calcium level at day 7 is higher in babies receiving breast milk than those receiving cows' milk (Oppé & Redstone, 1968). Knowing that cows' milk fat is poorly absorbed compared to that in breast milk fat, we might, wearing our 'blinkers', argue that these lower calcium concentrations were due to poorer absorption of cows' milk fat and, therefore, poorer absorption of calcium on cows' milk. There is indeed a poorer absorption of calcium but the serum calcium seems little to do with intestinal events; rather it is due to the ionic relationship between calcium and phosphorus. Babies receiving cows' milk have a higher intake of phosphorus, higher plasma phosphorus levels and, therefore, low concentrations of plasma calcium (Barltrop & Oppé, 1973). This is a well known example of how the plasma levels of two nutrients are affected more by the kidney and endocrine system than by the gastrointestinal tract. In a previously unexplored situation, however, the effects of factors outside the gastrointestinal tract may not be so immediately clear.

Urinary Excretion of Nutrients or their Products

Following the absorption of a varied diet and the interaction of the various substances which it contains, a proportion of the nutrients or their metabolites is incorporated into the tissues while the rest is excreted mainly in the urine, but also in sweat and also back into the gastrointestinal tract via bile and via exfoliation of cells.

Figure 2a illustrates these pathways in regard to protein nutrition. Apart from very small losses in the faeces and skin, most of the nitrogen leaving the body is in urine so that the absorbed nitrogen minus the urinary loss gives the apparent retention that is used for growth and general maintenance of tissues. When the protein intake is reduced urinary nitrogen falls by two possible mechanisms; either maintenance turnover remains constant and there is a change in the distribution of nitrogen so that a small proportion appears in the urine, Figure 2b, or the distribution remains constant and there is a reduction in maintenance turnover, Figure 2c. Amino acid turnover studies suggest that maintenance requirements remain constant (Waterlow & Stephen, 1967; Picou & Waterlow, 1968), and there is a reduction in the proportion of nitrogen excreted in the urine due to, or at least associated with, a reduction in the activity of the enzymes of the urea cycle (Schmike, 1962; Waterlow, 1968b). Exactly how a lowered nitrogen input causes the enzymes of the urea cycle to slow down is not fully understood. It takes about three days to do so in an adult man and may occur via an increase in growth hormone activity which inhibits certain enzymes of the urea cycle (McLean & Gurney, 1963).

In the newborn, therefore, the excretion of urea by a breast fed baby is considerably less than that by a baby on cows' milk who is receiving three times as much protein. In addition to these differences in nitrogen excretion of the newborn there are differences in mineral excretion too. Figure 3 shows the urinary constituents of babies receiving different milks and formulae. The baby receiving full cream cows' milk takes in more protein, calcium, phosphorus, sodium, etc. than one receiving breast milk. These extra nutrients are not required for growth or maintenance and so they, or their products are excreted in the urine, and so the total amount of solid in the urine of a baby receiving cows' milk is considerably higher than in the baby who is receiving breast milk, i.e. renal solute load of the diet is higher. The baby receiving unmodified cows' milk, therefore, produces a more concentrated urine, frequently has a high plasma osmolality and if he becomes dehydrated, say due to gastroenteritis, develops hyperosmolar dehydration which, in most series, has carried a higher mortality rate and a greater risk of neurological sequelae than is seen in infants with iso-osmolar dehydration (Finberg & Harrison, 1955; Macaulay & Watson, 1967). Figure 3 also shows how the renal solute load of cows' milk can be reduced by either adding carbohydrate (e.g. as in Ostermilk Complete, Cow and Gate Plus) or by using demineralised whey (e.g. 'S26' or Cow and Gate 'Premium').

69

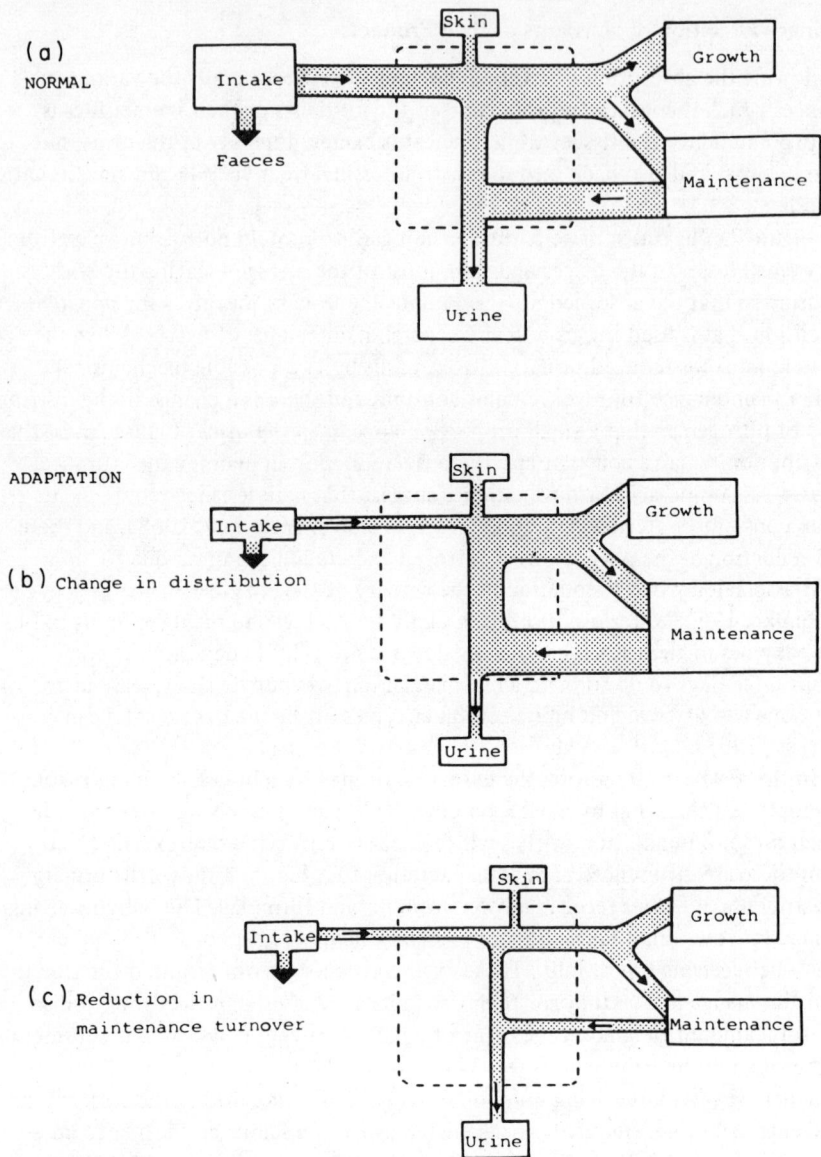

Figure 2. Possible mechanisms of adaptation to a low protein intake. The upper figure (a) shows general principles of nitrogen, balance and the two lower figures (b) and (c) both show the possible mechanisms resulting in a lower urinary nitrogen in response to a decreased protein intake (figure adapted and modified from Waterlow, 1968).

70

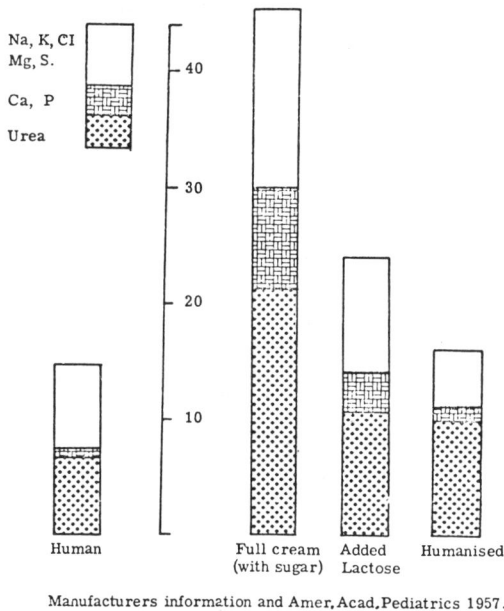

Na, K, Cl
Mg, S.

Ca, P

Urea

40

30

20

10

Human   Full cream   Added   Humanised
               (with sugar) Lactose

Manufacturers information and Amer.Acad.Pediatrics 1957.

Figure 3. Load of solutes requiring excretion when milk is fed to provide 130 kcal per kg day (units are in mosm per kg day).

Other dietary constituents may appear in urine and one of these is sulphur. Figure 4 shows the metabolism of the sulphur containing amino acids, methionine and cysteine. After absorption they may be used for the plasma proteins or new tissue, but if they are not required for protein synthesis then like any other amino acid they may be catabolised – the amino group producing urea. Catabolism of the sulphur-containing amino acids, particularly of cysteine also results in a release of sulphur. This is initially acidic and so can affect the acid base balance of the individual before it is buffered and excreted by the kidney as inorganic sulphate (Kildeburg & Winter, 1972). There is another pathway open to the sulphur-containing amino acids, however. Methionine may be converted to cysteine although in the early weeks of life a temporary deficiency of the liver enzyme cystathionase may limit this, possibly making cysteine an essential amino acid at this age (Gyorgy, 1971). Cysteine may then be converted to taurine which can conjugate with the bile acids and so appear in the bile. There is, therefore, this other excretory pathway apart from the kidney, to the bile. Most of this will then be re-cycled via the enterohepatic circulation, and other nutrients, e.g. B_{12} are re-cycled in a similar fashion. The excretion of nutrients by bile has perhaps not been studied as much as is necessary. Some of the trace elements are excreted in the bile and then partially re-absorbed, e.g. copper, so that in obstructive jaundice serum copper level usually rises. The excretion of certain trace elements in bile may account for the negative balance of these nutrients which occurs temporarily in the newborn (Widdowson, 1969).

71

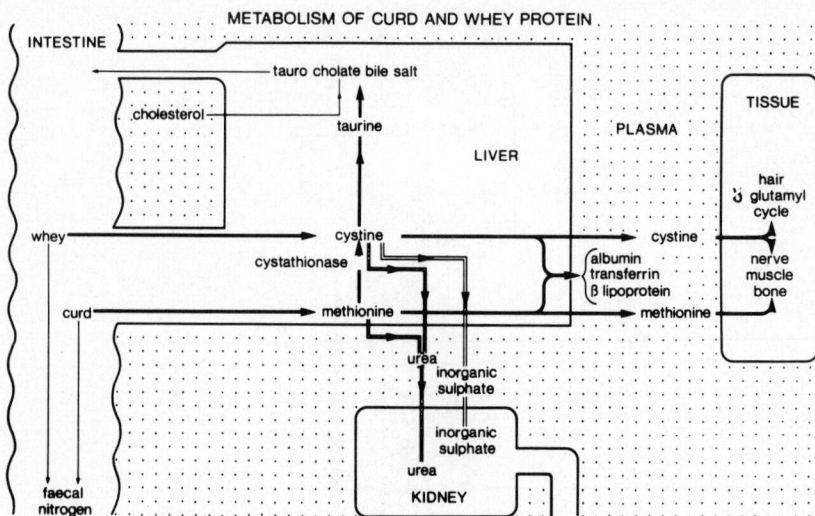

Figure 4. Possible metabolic pathways of the sulphur containing amino acids methionine, cysteine and taurine. (Note that cysteine is formed when 2 molecules of cysteine are reduced and linked by an -S-S-bond) — from Berger 1976.

Changes in Body Composition

Nutrients which are not excreted are retained and used either for maintenance of the existing tissues or for formation of new tissue, i.e. growth. The composition of these tissues, therefore, represents the balance of input minus losses. It is conceivable, therefore, that varied diets might result in varied body composition. The effect of variations in dietary protein and dietary fat on body composition have received some attention.

If we return to the differences in protein intake of babies receiving breast milk or cows' milk, although babies receiving cows' milk have higher urinary nitrogen levels this does not account for all the extra nitrogen absorbed; their apparent retention of nitrogen is still greater than in the breast fed babies. Since maintenance turnover is presumably similar in both groups it seems the extra protein retained by the cows' milk group is being laid down in the new tissues. Balance studies suggest that in the first 4 months of life 800 g of protein are laid down in the new tissue of the cows' milk fed child compared to only 400 g in the breast fed child, i.e. a divergence of body composition is occurring — the bottle fed baby is becoming older and more chemically mature. It seems, however, that these differences in calculated body composition, based on observations of apparent nitrogen retention, are due to the limitations of the nitrogen balance technique; errors such as small amounts of food being regurgitated, imperfect collection of urine and faeces, etc. exaggerate the apparent retention and the effect of these errors is proportionally greater in the diet containing the greater amount of protein (Wallace, 1959; Foman & Owen, 1962).

72

TABLE II. *Fatty Acid Composition of Adipose Tissue of British and Dutch Infants at 4 months of Life*

Fatty acid	Babies	
	British	Dutch
Linoleic acid 18:2	0–3%	32–37%
Myristic acid 14:0	8–10%	1–2%

Widdowson et al, 1975

Whether variations in the quantity of dietary protein affect body composition is, therefore, doubtful. On the other hand, variations in the quality of dietary fat do result in a definite alteration in body composition. In a number of infant feeding formulae the cows' milk fat has been replaced by oils. The choice of vegetable oil depends partly on commercial factors, but mainly on how well it is absorbed. Consequently oils, such as corn oil, have been used quite extensively and, for example in America and Europe, many formulae contain predominantly corn oil with little other fat. Table II shows the proportions of myristic and linoleic acid in the adipose tissue of British babies who mostly receive cows' milk fat and in Dutch babies receiving a corn oil formula. The composition of the body fat of British babies and the Dutch babies are quite different. In Dutch babies, a third of their adipose tissue when they were four months old consisted of linoleic acid; about twenty times as much as was found in the British babies (Widdowson et al, 1975). This may, or may not, be important, we do not know; however, polyunsaturated fatty acids, such as linoleic acid, when present in excess can cause problems, for example they increase the requirements for vitamin E (Harris & Embree, 1963). Vitamin E deficiency resulting in a syndrome of oedema, poor growth, haemolytic anaemia, and thrombocytosis has been described in premature babies receiving a diet rich in polyunsaturated fatty acids (Oski & Barness, 1965; Hassan et al, 1966).

The Final View

The fate of a feed, therefore, is as varied as the feed itself. Some nutrients begin or complete their action well before they are absorbed. In actual life nutrients act in concert; they may interact with each other as they are absorbed and as they are handled subsequently by the processes of intermediary metabolism. Urinary composition is a mirror of the diet, reflecting the adjustments and responses of the body to its very variable intake of nutrients. Finally, although different patterns of feeding may result in quantitative and qualitative differences in body composition, perhaps the remarkable thing is that such differences are not much wider than they in fact are.

73

References

Barltrop, D and Oppé, T D (1973) *Archives of Disease in Childhood, 48,* 580

Berger, H M (1976) *M.D. thesis submitted to University of Birmingham*

Bullen, C L & Willis, A T (1971) *British Medical Journal, 3,* 338

Bullen, J J, Rogers, Henry J & Leigh, L (1972) *British Medical Journal, 3,* 69

Cook, G C (1974) *Gut, 15,* 239

DHSS (1974) *Present-day practice in infant feeding.* Report on Health and Social Subjects No.9, London, HMSO. Page 7

Finberg, L & Harrison, H G (1955) *Pediatrics, 16,* 1

Foman, S J & Owen, G M (1962) *Pediatrics, 29,* 495

Gerstley, J R, Cohn, D J & Lawrence G (1945) *Journal of Paediatrics, 27,* 521

Greenwald, E, Samachson, J & Spencer, H (1963) *Journal of Nutrition, 79,* 531

Gyorgy, P (1971) *American Journal of Clinical Nutrition, 24,* 970

Harris, P L & Embree, N D (1963) *American Journal of Clinical Nutrition, 13,* 385

Hassan, H T, Hashim, S A, von Itallie, T B and Sebrell, W H (1966) *American Journal of Clinical Nutrition, 19,* 147

Kenny, J F, Boesman, M I, Michaels, R H (1967) *Pediatrics, 39,* 202

Kildeburg, P and Winters, R (1972) *Pediatrics, 49,* 801

Macaulay, D and Watson, M (1967) *Archives of Disease in Childhood, 42,* 485

McLean, P and Gurney, M W (1963) *Biochemical Journal, 87,* 96

Mills, R, Breiter, H, Kempster, E, McKey, B, Pickens, M & Outhouse, J (1940) *Journal of Nutrition, 20,* 467

Nutrition Society (1973) *Symposium on Fibre in Human Nutrition. Proceedings of the Nutrition Society, 32,* 123

Oppé, T E and Redstone, D (1968) *Lancet, i,* 1045

Oski, F A and Barness, L A (1965) *Journal of Pediatrics, 67,* 1045

Picou, D and Waterlow, J C (1968) *Amino Acid Metabolism and Genetic Variation* (Ed.) W L Nyhan. McGraw-Hill, London. Page 421

Rossiter, M A, Palmer, T, Evans, K and Wharton, B A (1974) *British Journal of Nutrition, 32,* 605

Schmike, R T (1962) *Journal of Biological Chemistry, 237,* 1921

Schulz, S G & Curran, P F (1970) *Physiological Review, 50,* 637

Wallace, W M (1959) *Federated Proceedings, 18,* 1125

Waterlow, J C and Stephen, J M L (1967) *Clinical Science, 33,* 489

Waterlow, J C (1968a) *Lancet, ii,* 1091

Waterlow, J C (1968b) *Protein Deficiencies and Calorie Deficiencies.* (Eds) R A McCance and E M Widdowson. Churchill, London, Page 61

Widdowson, E M (1969) *Mineral Metabolism in Paediatrics.* (Ed) D Barltrop and W L Burland. Blackwell, Oxford. Page 85

Widdowson, E M, Dauncey, M J, Gairdner, D M T, Jonxis, J H P, and Pelikan-Filipkova, M (1975) *British Medical Journal, 1,* 653

Discussion

DR MOWAT Dr Wharton, the immunoglobulins and lactoferrin which prevent bacterial growth, are these substances heat stable? I am really thinking of the breast milk which we tend to dispense to young infants after pasteurisation.

WHARTON Biochemically, if you pasteurise breast milk by the most common pasteurisation processes you will certainly precipitate, or at least alter, the electrophoretic mobility of lactoferrin so that in all probability it has been denatured, and so has the IgA. Having said that, however, I think that Dr Dolby, at Northwick Park, nevertheless still shows that pasteurised breast milk does have some antibacterial activity.

PROFESSOR HADORN I have been very interested by the remark that the iron you give will neutralise the lactoferrin. Would it be possible to make a study in which one compares children, neonates or even prematures, who have received iron with those who have not received iron, to see if those who have received iron have more infections?

WHARTON One snag about a lot of this is that you can show what happens *in vitro* and then you show what happens *in vivo* in animals, and also in humans, but then the final step, showing epidemiologically what is important in thousands of babies, is often missing. I do not know of any work saying it is specifically iron. It may also be that the iron is absorbed because it saturates transferrin which is essentially the same protein, and that when in the circulation it may affect protection against bacteria. There is a little bit more evidence on this, that giving Imferon, for example, does make children susceptible.

DR McNEISH Dr Wharton started by saying that children throughout the world have remarkably different diets and yet finish remarkably similarly. Dr Widdowson, with her animal studies, and Dr Ounsted in the 'Lancet' recently, are both drawing our attention to the general phenomenon of babies tending towards the mean, perhaps because of appetite. They eat what they need. I wondered if you could extend that sort of observation to take account of the eating, not just the diet that is on the table, but the actual eating habits of infants and children. Do you think that this is correct, that children tend to eat what they require?

WHARTON I really do not know. There is another big variation which could be a control factor which I have not mentioned, and that is variation in activity. Certainly studies of physical activity in children who are not on an absolutely optimal diet does suggest that their activity reduces very, very considerably and that therefore this may be a very substantial saving on calories.

DR DODGE It is worthwhile keeping in mind the fact that composition of breast milk varies from the beginning to the end of the feed and when the baby stops feeding it can possibly be because of a change in the milk. This may be yet another variable to consider along with his basic appetite.

WHARTON The variation in the composition of breast milk is both a diurnal variation, and, as you say, the breast milk varies during the course of the feed. It also varies according to the stage of lactation, and the mother's diet and so on. When you look at the published figures on the composition of breast milk, the actual number of breast milk compositions we have analysed is very small.

DR D P DAVIES   What do you think the effect of mother's diet is, particularly on the pattern of fatty acids?

WHARTON   Certainly the pattern of the mother's diet in respect of fatty acids is reflected in her milk. For example, I think in Tanzania, some women have about 18% of polyunsaturated fatty acids in their breast milk, whereas in Europe it mostly runs at about 8% and does not seem to get much lower. Therefore, what the mother eats will certainly affect the fat that the baby deposits post-natally. Whether the diet that she has ante-natally, as regards fatty acids, affects the *fetus* is a different matter. The work that Dr Widdowson did with people from Holland showed that there was a tendency for the Dutch babies *at birth,* before they had been fed, to have more unsaturated fatty acids in their fat (Widdowson et al, 1975). You may have seen the letter that we published in the 'British Medical Journal' about this (Fosbrooke & Wharton, 1975). The fat composition of babies in London was like Dutch babies, not like Cambridge babies at all. We began to think the mothers in the East End must have large amounts of unsaturated fatty acids. We thought the differences were methodological, but we may be wrong. If you feed guinea pigs a lot of polyunsaturated fatty acids, then the baby guinea pigs at birth have a lot of polyunsaturated fatty acids in their depot fat, so that if the human is behaving like a guinea pig, perhaps there is something in it.

References

Fosbrooke, A and Wharton, B (1975) *British Medical Journal, 2,* 616
Widdowson, E M, Dauncey, M J, Gairdner, D M T, Jonxis, J H P and Pelikan-Filípková, M (1975) *British Medical Journal, 1,* 653

The Mechanism of Vomiting

B W LAWRIE

Vomiting has been defined by Borison and Wang (1953) as forceful expulsion of gastrointestinal contents through the mouth. Retching is defined as laboured rhythmical activity of the respiratory musculature which usually precedes or accompanies vomiting. Vomiting is not invariably a consequence of retching.

Vomiting is a highly integrated, chiefly somatic act. This has been shown by the fact that denervation of the gastrointestinal tract produces no essential differences in the characteristics of vomiting, compared with that of the intact animal (Hatcher, 1924). During vomiting the gastric contents are expelled through the relaxed oesophagus and open mouth by contraction of the abdominal and thoracic musculature. The only portion of the stomach which is contracted is the pyloric end, whereas the rest of the stomach is in a relaxed state. The nasal and pharyngeal air passages are occluded by elevation of the soft palate and closure of the glottis with forward movement of the larynx and hyoid bone.

McCarthy and his colleagues recently studied the emetic process by correlating radiology, intrathoracic and intra-abdominal pressure changes, and EMG activity of the diaphragm during vomiting in the decerebrate cat. They showed that during a single emetic episode there were repeated negative thoracic and coincidental positive abdominal pressure pulses, which coincided radiographically with the rapid descent of the diaphragm which engulfed the fundus of the stomach and abolished the intra-abdominal portion of the oesophagus. With each repetition of this cycle there was reflux of gastric contents into the oesophagus with the formation of a sliding hiatus hernia. When expulsion occurred this was characterised by a positive thoracic pressure pulse which distinguished the preceding retching from the vomiting which then occurred. At this point the diaphragm ascended rapidly without the stomach returning to the abdomen and the compression of the herniated stomach was accompanied by the expulsion of the vomitus (McCarthy et al, 1974).

Central control of vomiting is very complex, but basically there are two areas in the medulla which control or initiate the act of vomiting. The so-called *vomiting centre* is found in the region of the medulla corresponding to the fasciculus solitarius and an adjacent portion of the lateral reticular formation. It is situated close to other medullary centres concerned with sporadic respiration, inspiratory and expiratory centres, the vasomotor centre, the salivatory nuclei, vestibular nuclei and the bulbofacilitatory and inhibitory systems (Borison & Wang, 1953). The vomiting centre cannot be sharply or geometrically circumscribed, but it co-ordinates and integrates the activities of the neuronal structures in its vicinity to produce the complex act of vomiting. It may be activated by afferent impulses from the gut or by impulses from higher centres of the brain. The second important area is the *chemoreceptive trigger zone* which lies in the floor of the fourth ventricle corresponding to the area postrema, which is an ependymal layer. This trigger zone is sensitive to emetic chemicals such as apomorphine, but is not excited by electrical stimulation, and has been shown to be an afferent station for the vomiting centre. It has no integral part in the control of vomiting and cannot produce vomiting without an intact vomiting centre (Borison & Wang, 1953). The main efferent fibres concerned with vomiting are carried in the phrenic nerves, spinal nerves and special efferent fibres from the vagus to the voluntary muscles of the larynx and pharynx as vomiting is a chiefly somatic muscle process.

References

Borison, H L and Wang, S C (1953). *Pharmacological Reviews, 5,* 193
Hatcher, R A (1949) *Physiological Reviews, 4,* 479
McCarthy, L E, Borison, H L, Spiegel, P K and Friedlander, R N (1974) *Gastroenterology, 67,* 1126
Wang, S C and Borison, H L (1952) *Gastroenterology, 22,* 1

The Vomiting Infant

J A DODGE

Vomiting of mild degree is sufficiently common in early infancy to be regarded as a normal feature of behaviour. Thus Shakespeare described the infant 'mewling and puking in the nurse's arms'. It is precisely this fact — that the mother's anatomy or clothing may be the target for the liquid assault — which brings some infants to medical attention. In these cases, sympathy and reassurance are all that is required, because the babies are thriving, the symptoms are mild, and the clothes can be dry-cleaned. It is nevertheless difficult to define the boundary between acceptable regurgitation and pathological vomiting, because sometimes an infant with a definite anatomical lesion may have grown well despite his symptom, or maternal concern may be inappropriately low.

I shall attempt to define some of the clinical features and diagnostic procedures related to vomiting in the first year of life, before discussing some specific disorders in greater detail. The clinical approach is determined to some extent by the age of the baby. During the first week obstructive lesions of the alimentary tract must be considered, and persistent vomiting is also a feature of some inborn metabolic errors. Infection of the meninges or urinary tract may also present in this way. I shall discuss the self-limiting early neonatal vomiting of mucus again when we consider peptic ulcers, because I believe that this symptom may denote acute gastritis associated with disturbed acid secretion and the stress of birth. After the first week, congenital obstructive malformations are less likely to present for the first time, but pyloric stenosis needs to be considered more seriously and so does hiatus hernia (partial thoracic stomach). The inspissated milk syndrome characteristically occurs between 3 and 14 days, but may be later in pre-term infants. 'Feeding problems' are likely to appear during the first month of life. This description may be applied to infants whose vomiting clears up at once on admission to hospital without special treatment, and where the mother may be over-anxious, inexperienced, rejecting, or just inadequate. Sometimes there is a deep-seated abnormality of the mother–child relationship, but more often the vomiting and maternal anxiety form a vicious circle, which can be broken by the intervention of sympathetic and supportive nursing staff. Diagnoses to be considered in babies whose vomiting begins after the first month include subdural haematoma, idiopathic hypercalcaemia,

79

and food intolerances, particularly to cow's milk protein. Not uncommonly the latter condition presents as vomiting which starts when the infant is weaned from the breast (Table I).

TABLE I. Causes of Vomiting in Infancy *and Childhood*

---

functional

DIGESTIVE TRACT DISORDERS

Idiopathic Neonatal Vomiting	1
Idiopathic Infantile Vomiting ('Pylorospasm')	(1), 2, 3, (1)
Feeding Problems ('Rumination', i.e., abnormal mother–child relationship)	2, 3

Cyclical vomiting. 4

Malformations and obstructions

Hiatus Hernia and Gastro-oesophageal reflux	2, 1, 3, 4
Gastric outlet malformation	1, (2), 3, 4
Pyloric stenosis	(1), 2, 3, (1)
Volvulus: gastric or intestinal	1, 2, 3, 4
Malrotation and partial obstructions	1, 2, 3, 4
Atresias	1
Meconium ileus *← intestinal obstruction syndrome (meconium ileus equivalent)*	1 4
Distal → Inspissated milk syndrome *and lactobezoar* 4	1, 2
Duplications	1, 2, 3, 4
Intusussusception	3
Aganglionic megacolon (Hirschsprung's disease)	1, 2, (3)
Peptic ulcer	1, 2, 3

Trichobezoar 4

Food Intolerances

Coeliac disease	3
Cow's milk protein intolerance	3, (2)
Other food intolerances	3

INFECTIVE DISORDERS

Gastroenteritis	1, 2, 3, 4
Epidemic vomiting	3, 4
Thrush	1, 2
Urinary tract infection *(also hydronephrosis and renal calculi)*	1, 2, 3, 4
Respiratory tract infection *(including otitis)*	1, 2, 3, 4
Appendicitis *(and other surgical emergencies)*	3, 4

NEUROLOGICAL

CEREBRAL DISORDERS

Meningitis and encephalitis	1, 2, 3, 4
Intracranial birth injury	1

Migraine 4

Increased Intracranial Pressure

Hydrocephalus	1, 2, 3, 4
Subdural haematoma	(1), 2, 3, (1), 4
Tumour, including diencephalic syndrome	3, 4
Hypertension	(2), 3, (2), 4
Kernicterus	1, 2

Motion sickness (4)

80

(TABLE I. Causes of Vomiting in Infancy — continued)

TOXIC/METABOLIC DISORDERS	2,
Adrenal hyperplasia	2, 1, 3
Phenylketonuria	1, 2
Galactosaemia	1, 2
Hypercalcaemia	3, 4
Uraemia	1, 2, 3, 4
Neonatal Cold Injury	1
Drugs, e.g. Digoxin, *cytotoxic agents, anticonvulsic*	1, 2, 3, 4
Vitamin A excess	3
Diabetes mellitus (ketoacidosis)	4
too many ***Hepatic Disorders***	
Hepatitis syndrome	1, 2, 3
Cardiac failure	1, 2, 3
Exchange Transfusion — *Reye's syndrome*	1 (3), 4

Key: 1 = First week; 2 = 1 week to 1 month; 3 = 1 month to 1 year   *4 = over 1 year*

CLINICAL FEATURES

History

The time of vomiting in relation to feeding may give some indication of the site of the problem, but it is not often very helpful in this age group. Of greater help is a description of the contents of the vomitus: was the volume greater than one feed, did it smell sour, did it contain blood, coffee-grounds material, bile or mucus? Projectile vomiting, described with the typical 'pyloric gesture', occurs in hiatus hernia and adrenal hyperplasia as well as in pyloric stenosis and duodenal atresia, but it makes a test feed mandatory. The mother may have noticed that changes in posture affect the frequency and severity of the vomiting, and this feature is important because it may suggest hiatus hernia or gastric volvulus. Other symptoms which should be enquired about include diarrhoea, constipation, and jaundice. Of course, the health of other family members and recent contacts is also very relevant.

Examination

During the standard clinical assessment of a vomiting baby, particular attention should be paid to examination of the mouth for thrush, and for signs of dehydration. Jaundice should lead to a consideration of hepatitis, urinary tract infection, malformations such as choledochal cyst or biliary atresia, and upper alimentary obstruction. A tense fontanelle suggests meningitis, cerebral tumour, hydrocephalus, hypercalcaemia or vitamin A intoxication. Arterial

81

hypertension occurs in some renal and suprarenal disorders which may present with vomiting, and in coarctation of the aorta — one of the causes of cardiac failure in infancy, which itself may produce vomiting as a result of gastric and hepatic venous engorgement.

In the abdomen, the presence and location of distension should be noted, as well as visible peristalsis, and alterations in bowel sounds. The size of palpable organs, the presence of abnormal masses, and areas of tenderness or guarding will of course be evident on routine examination.

A test feed, with palpation for a pyloric tumour, will often be required, and this is best performed after the stomach has been emptied either by vomiting or via an intragastric catheter. It has been suggested that intermittent aspiration during the course of a test feed will prevent distension of the stomach and make it easier to feel the pylorus (Toyama, 1969). One negative feed test does not exclude pyloric stenosis, and the examination may need to be repeated on more than one occasion.

If the child is in hospital, nursing staff should be asked to record intake of feeds, urinary output, volume, frequency and timing of vomiting in relation to feeds, the presence of blood, mucus or bile, and the frequency, character and volume of stools.

Investigations

As a routine, vomiting babies will require side-room analysis of the urine for protein, blood, bile, acetone and reducing substances, and in some cases laboratory analysis of amino acids. Laboratory cultures of urine and stools, and examination of the urinary deposit should be performed on all infants. The blood should be analysed for urea and electrolytes, calcium and phosphorus, and acid-base status. A plain x-ray of the abdomen, in supine and erect postures, is necessary if obstruction is under consideration, and unexpected intrathoracic lesions such as cardiac malformations or diaphragmatic hernia occur sufficiently often to make a routine chest x-ray worthwhile. In most cases, a barium meal will be required, and there is no doubt that the value of this investigation is greatly determined by the experience and interest of the radiologist. I shall return to this theme later. Although we are not especially concerned with haematemesis, if large amounts of blood are present, then upper alimentary endoscopy may be a valuable diagnostic procedure. Other investigations, related to possible diagnoses outside the alimentary tract, such as lumbar puncture or intravenous pyelography, may be suggested by the clinical findings.

In practice, most conditions causing vomiting in the first week of life are readily diagnosed, but there remains a large group of infants with persistent vomiting who may need repeated radiological studies and in whom the diagnosis lies between hiatus hernia, pyloric stenosis, vomiting of unknown cause, and, occasionally, cow's milk protein intolerance. It is these conditions which I would like to consider in greater detail.

HIATUS HERNIA (PARTIAL THORACIC STOMACH)

The many different names given to this condition are an indication of the confusion which has existed about its true nature. Table II is taken from a recent American paper and it lists some of the synonyms used on both sides of the Atlantic (Darling et al, 1974). The most widely used description in this country is 'hiatus hernia', but perhaps the most satisfactory is 'partial thoracic stomach' because it simply states an anatomical fact without implying an aetiology.

Table II. Terminology

Partial thoracic stomach
Sliding (axial) hiatus hernia
Congenitally short oesophagus
Incompetence of the gastric cardia
Gastro-oesophageal relaxation
Cardio-oesophageal relaxation
Cardio-oesophageal syndrome
Lax oesophagus
Chalasia

(Darling, Fisher & Gellis, 1974)

Incidence

Until recently, it was believed that hiatus hernia was commoner in the UK than in North America, and various theories were advanced to explain the discrepancy. One of the most plausible was the observation that American practice is to nurse infants in the prone position, which reduces the tendency to gastro-oesophageal reflux and would therefore prevent milder cases becoming manifest. It was shown by Friedland et al (1974) that the incidence of hiatus hernia in infants in their unit at Stanford University increased eleven-fold when they introduced diagnostic criteria used at the Hospital for Sick Children, Great Ormond Street, and Darling's group reported a similar experience from Boston. In the current Yearbook of Paediatrics, Gellis concludes that 'there are no striking differences in the prevalence of infantile hiatal hernia, but there are differences in the techniques used by radiologists to diagnose the disorder . . . I believe that we and others in the United States have missed the diagnosis in the past, and that we are not presently overdiagnosing.' (Gellis, 1975).

If this is the true state of affairs, then the likely incidence in British (and probably most European) centres should be similar to that found by Carré in Birmingham and in Northern Ireland, i.e. about 1 in 1,000 live births (Carré, 1975a). It is quite evident from the experience of colleagues in several British centres that there is still a great deal of variation in the frequency with which the diagnosis is made, and it seems highly probable that cases are being missed in centres with an apparently low incidence.

83

Pathophysiology

Most authors agree that the infantile form of hiatus hernia is a congenital malformation. Familial cases occur, and in these instances the mode of inheritance
is autosomal dominant. Asymptomatic hiatal herniae sometimes occur, without
gastro-oesophageal reflux, but the majority of patients with reflux have an
associated partial thoracic stomach. It seems therefore that the intrathoracic
location of the gastro-oesophageal sphincter is an important factor in producing
reflux. A sphincter situated normally in the abdomen has only to protect the
oesophagus against pressure changes generated within the stomach itself; but
when it is displaced, into the thorax, it may be inadequate to resist the combined
force of intragastric changes and the difference between intra-abdominal and
intrathoracic pressures. Under resting conditions this pressure difference varies
from 1 to 15 mmHg and is modified by posture, but deep inspiration, coughing,
or straining at stool cause a considerable further discrepancy. When there is
free communication between the intrathoracic and abdominal portions of the
stomach, the pressure in the thoracic loculus is the same as that in the remainder, derived from general intra-abdominal pressure and intragastric tension, but
the sphincter has only the lower — and variable — intrathoracic surrounding
pressure to support its attempts at competence. This mechanical disadvantage
is independent of the size of the gastric loculus, and indeed it is common
experience that infants with small herniae often have the most severe symptoms.

Reflux of gastric secretions into the oesophagus leads to inflammation,
bleeding, ulceration, and sometimes fibrosis with formation of a stricture. The
oesophageal mucosa is lined with squamous, not columnar epithelium, and the
transition is clearly seen during oesophagoscopy. When strictures occur, they
do so usually but not always at this junction. The object of management is to
prevent oesophagitis, and especially to avoid stricture formation, which,
although uncommon, is a medical disaster.

Clinical Features

Vomiting starting shortly after birth is the usual mode of presentation. It is
frequently projectile, and intermittently bloodstained, although major haematemesis is not commonly due to hiatus hernia. Continued occult bleeding sometimes leads to anaemia even in the absence of vomiting. Mucus and occasionally
bile may be present in the vomitus.

If the vomiting is severe, the infant fails to thrive. Dehydration may occur,
as in pyloric stenosis, which is the most important differential diagnosis. The
two conditions occur together about ten times as often as would be expected
by chance (Figure 1); a combination known as Roviralta's syndrome (Roviralta,
1950). Another eponym records Sandifer's observation that some older
children with hiatus hernia adopt bizarre postures of the head and neck, presumably as an anti-reflux measure.

Recurrent aspiration pneumonia is an obvious hazard of continued vomiting,
and is sometimes the presenting feature in older infants.

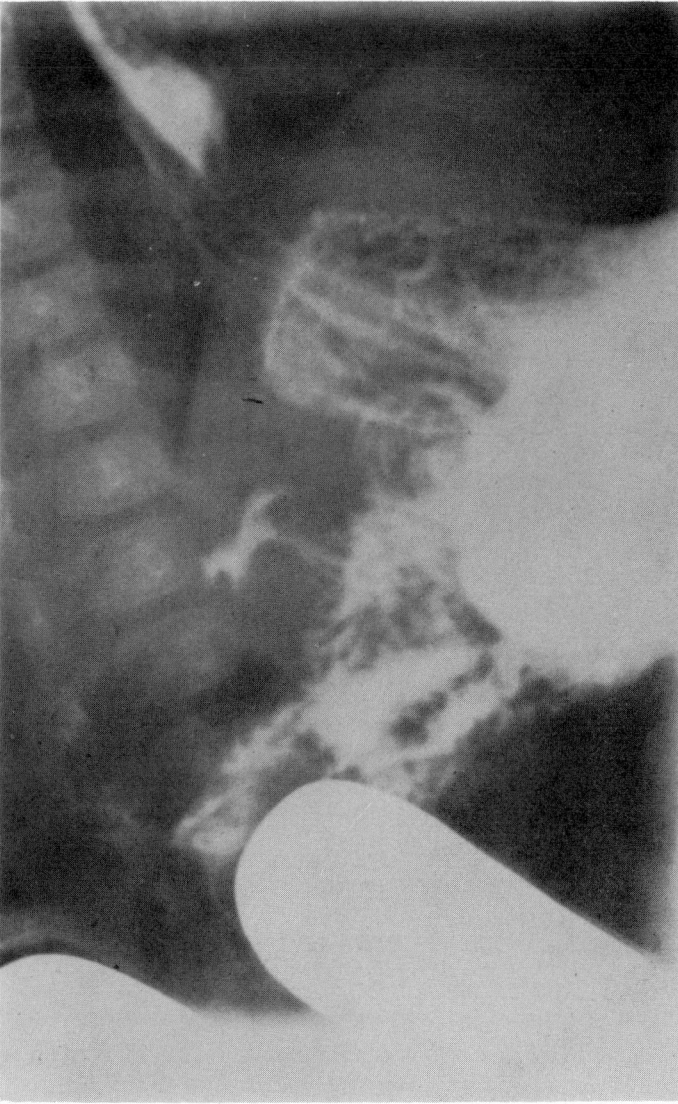

Figure 1. Roviralta Syndrome: Hiatus hernia and hypertrophic pyloric stenosis.

The symptoms usually improve without any special treatment when solid food is introduced into the diet, but this spontaneous 'cure' can be speeded up by keeping the infant propped up in a chair, night and day, as soon as the diagnosis is made. Only a small proportion of untreated patients (5%) will go on to develop strictures, but it is not possible to predict the outcome with any accuracy except insofar as failure of the symptoms to resolve on weaning may be regarded as a warning sign. There is no correlation between gastric acid output and the occurrence of strictures (Lari & Lister, 1972). The natural history of partial thoracic stomach has been authoritatively described by Carré (1959), and is summarized in Figure 2.

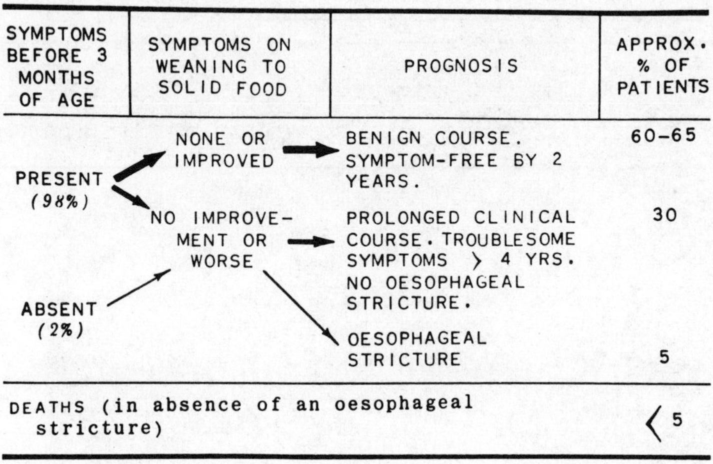

SYMPTOMS BEFORE 3 MONTHS OF AGE	SYMPTOMS ON WEANING TO SOLID FOOD	PROGNOSIS	APPROX. % OF PATIENTS
PRESENT (98%)	NONE OR IMPROVED	BENIGN COURSE. SYMPTOM-FREE BY 2 YEARS.	60–65
	NO IMPROVEMENT OR WORSE	PROLONGED CLINICAL COURSE. TROUBLESOME SYMPTOMS > 4 YRS. NO OESOPHAGEAL STRICTURE.	30
ABSENT (2%)		OESOPHAGEAL STRICTURE	5
DEATHS (in absence of an oesophageal stricture)			< 5

Figure 2. The Natural History of Partial Thoracic Stomach (From Carré, 1959, used by permission of the author)

Radiological Features

The radiological criteria described by Chrispin and Friedland (1967) have recently been expanded and validated in Friedland's series (Table III). The characteristic features relate to the intrathoracic location of the gastro-oesophageal sphincter. The vestibule is seen to close, even briefly, between the oesophagus above and a gastric loculus (pouchlike or sometimes tubelike) below, and it opens on deglutition: either a 'dry' swallow or a bolus of barium. The diaphragm is seen to compress the stomach as it passes from abdomen to thorax. Other useful features include the presence of thick gastric rugae lining the thoracic stomach, and the lack of peristalsis in the gastric loculus. Free gastro-oesophageal reflux is seen, particularly with small herniae, and there may be evidence of oesophagitis (Friedland et al, 1974).

86

The importance of screening by a skilled radiologist is evident, and the value of 'spot' films is limited. As with so many other conditions, those who seek shall find.

TABLE III. Features of Hiatal Hernia in Infants and Children (Friedland et al, 1974)

Characteristic x-ray features
Vestibule closes between the barium filled oesophageal body above and herniated tubular pouchlike stomach below
Vestibule opens on deglutition – either a 'dry' swallow or swallowed bolus
Diaphragm compresses stomach at hiatus as it passes from abdomen to thorax

Other x-ray features
Numerous thick folds, which have a rugal pattern, line the intrathoracic gastric loculus
Intrathoracic gastric loculus lacks peristaltic activity
Thoracic loculus expands during inspiration
Abnormally long 'vestibule'
Free gastro-oesophageal reflux
Features of oesophagitis
Motility disturbances
Asperistalsis
Single or repetitive nonperistaltic contractions
Atony and dilatation (megaoesophagus)
Irregular luminal contour; oesophageal wall thickening
Luminal narrowing
Reversible, due to oedema or spasm
Persistent, due to fibrous stricture

Management

Postural treatment with the infant propped up at a minimum angle of 60° from the horizontal is the most effective anti-reflux manoeuvre and should be continued until the infant has been symptom free for at least six weeks. A minority of patients respond only slowly to this regime, particularly when treatment has been delayed until late infancy. Adjuncts to postural treatment, particularly indicated when response is slow, include thickening of the feeds with 'Nestargel' and the use of antacids to minimise the risk of oesophagitis. Metoclopramide might be expected to help but has not been widely used.

The place of surgery is very uncertain. A variety of different procedures has been used, with very mixed reported results. The excellent results of postural therapy, the rarity of strictures, and the difficulty in predicting their formation, means that surgical treatment in cases uncomplicated by stricture should be reserved for those infants where no response to postural treatment has occurred after a minimum of three months, and it should rarely be considered before the age of one year (Carré, 1975b). Where surgery is undertaken, the Nissen type of fundoplication, which retains the gastro-oesophageal sphincter within a sleeve of gastric fundus, is the operation of choice. Radiological appearances of oesophageal narrowing can be produced by local inflammatory oedema and spasm, and may resolve without surgical intervention. Established fibrous stricture may require resection and insertion of a colonic transplant, but conservative treatment with repeated dilatation should first be tried, and is often sufficient (Lister & Wright, 1967). In 83 infants with a combination of reflux and pyloric stenosis (some of whom had demonstrated partial thoracic stomach), the reflux usually disappeared within a few months of pyloromyotomy (Pellerin et al, 1974).

Prognosis

Although 95% of patients will eventually lose their symptoms without special treatment (and much more rapidly if given postural therapy) only about a third have a radiological cure. The remainder retain their intrathoracic loculus of stomach, but enjoy normal health (Carré & Astley, 1960). Whether they will have a recurrence of symptoms in middle age is unknown.

INFANTILE PYLORIC STENOSIS

It has been my impression, and that of colleagues in other centres, that pyloric stenosis in babies is becoming less common. The reason for this decrease is not very clear, but the whole aetiology of this condition is shrouded in mystery. It is evident that it is not a true congenital malformation, but an acquired lesion — acquired either in late pregnancy or early postnatal life. There are, fortunately, few problems of diagnosis, and none of management, so my discussion will be limited to some observations about the aetiology and pathogenesis and to some of the complications.

Aetiology

A genetic predisposition to the development of pyloric hypertrophy has been noted by many authors, but although striking aggregations of cases occur in some families with as many as five consecutive sibs affected, the genetics do not follow Mendelian principles. The striking male preponderance, about 4:1 cannot be entirely explained by X-linkage, although it is possible that an X-linked gene may play a contributory role in some cases. There is evidence that

88

pyloric stenosis may be even commoner in XO Turner's syndrome females than in males (Benson & King, 1964). The largest genetic study was that of Carter and Evans (1969) from London. These authors concluded that the genetic basis was provided by multiple genes, and the condition appears only when the genetic 'load' crosses a threshold of expression. This threshold is set at a higher level for females, who therefore require a greater genetic load before they express the disease. Such a hypothesis explains the common observation that relatives of affected females, especially male relatives, are particularly likely to be affected themselves, because the female patient with her heavy 'load' of contributory genes will share them with her relatives, and the males will require a smaller 'load' before they are affected. In general, my own series of 480 patients from Belfast supported the observations of Carter and Evans and in both centres the heritability for first degree relatives was of the order of 80%. In an attempt to define some of the relevant genes, I looked at the ABO blood groups of the Belfast patients and found a marked lack of Group A. Surprisingly, this deficiency of Group A was even more striking in the *mothers* of affected infants (Dodge, 1973). In a smaller series in Cardiff, we have not been able to confirm this abnormal blood group distribution, nor have we yet found any abnormality of the HL-A antigens (Orellana et al, 1975).

The fact that pyloric stenosis sometimes appears in only one of identical twins highlights the importance of non-genetic factors in its aetiology. The first born preponderance clearly seen in some series but not in others, is another facet which cannot be explained on a genetic basis. A high incidence of maternal stress in the latter part of pregnancy has been reported (Dodge, 1972) and confirmed in a recent study which is still in progress. We found that stressful life events, defined and given heavy weighting by groups of psychiatrists, students and patients, occurred with increased frequency in the last trimester of pregnancy of 80 women giving birth to infants with pyloric stenosis. The controls were a group of 60 unselected 'normal' women giving birth to healthy babies (Revill & Dodge 1975). Further unpublished observations have shown that mothers of infants with a true congenital malformation, spina bifida, also report significantly fewer stressful events in pregnancy than the mothers of the pylorics. It is possible that the anxiety and emotional disturbances provoked by stress may have biochemical consequences which affect the fetal stomach and initiate pyloric hypertrophy. If so, it might be possible to reproduce the disease in experimental animals by giving an appropriate physiological stimulant to the fetal pylorus by way of the maternal circulation.

Such an experiment has been attempted, using pentagastrin as the biochemical mediator, and proved successful in inducing pyloric tumour formation in some pups of two bitches who were given the pentagastrin by depot injections during the last few weeks of pregnancy (Dodge, 1970). This work has been repeated in a larger series by Mr Ali Karim, with varying degrees of success. It appears that some animals are more susceptible than others to equivalent doses of pentagastrin, just as in the human situation. In some cases, good pyloric tumours were produced in the pups, but in others the pentagastrin seemed to have little effect (Karim et al, 1974). As one would expect, some of the puppies also acquired peptic ulcers — found in the duodenum, prepyloric region and the oesophagus.

Karim further showed that ganglion cell changes, described in infantile pyloric stenosis but of uncertain significance, were present in puppies with pentagastrin-induced tumours, and that pyloric motility was disorganised in affected animals (Karim, 1975). It seems therefore that this is a valid animal model, but of course this does not mean that gastrin is necessarily involved in producing the human disorder. We know that gastrin crosses the placenta in dogs, and probably in humans, but the newborn infant also produces endogenous gastrin (Rogers et al, 1974) and continue to do so with higher serum levels than adults throughout the first year of life (Becker et al, 1975). Fasting plasma gastrin levels in 14 affected infants were found by Rogers and his co-workers to be similar to those of controls. No significant difference was found in the mean fasting gastric pH although greater volumes of gastric juice were observed in affected babies. These authors suggested that infants with pyloric stenosis may have a higher parietal cell mass than normals, with resultant increased acid secretion prior to developing pyloric tumours. They speculated that cholecystokinin and secretin, released in response to gastric hyperacidity, may act as an hormonal drive to pyloric contraction and stimulate circular muscle hypertrophy (Figure 3). They point out that both pyloric stenosis and duodenal ulcer have a male preponderance, and noted the association between ulceration and pyloric hypertrophy in some of the experimental animals (Rogers et al, 1975). A similar association has been observed in a number of infants, and an increased incidence of ulcers in later life in the survivors of Ramstedt's operation has also been reported. In 8 patients where acid secretion was estimated before Ramstedt's operation, I found basal output to be above normal in 4 and peak output above normal in 2, whereas postoperative secretion was in the normal range for both basal and peak output in all but 2 (Dodge, 1971a — Figure 4).

Family histories of 'peptic' ulcer were consistently more frequent for all grades of relationship when 475 children with a history of infantile pyloric stenosis were compared with 181 control children of similar age. Ulcers occurred in 14 control fathers (7.7%) but in 55 'pyloric' fathers (11.6%). This difference was statistically significant. There was also a markedly higher incidence of undiagnosed ulcer-type dyspepsia in fathers of affected babies (Dodge, 1971b). These observations perhaps support the suggestion that acid hypersecretion may be a precursor of pyloric hypertrophy, and that there are close similarities between infantile pyloric stenosis and adult duodenal ulcer.

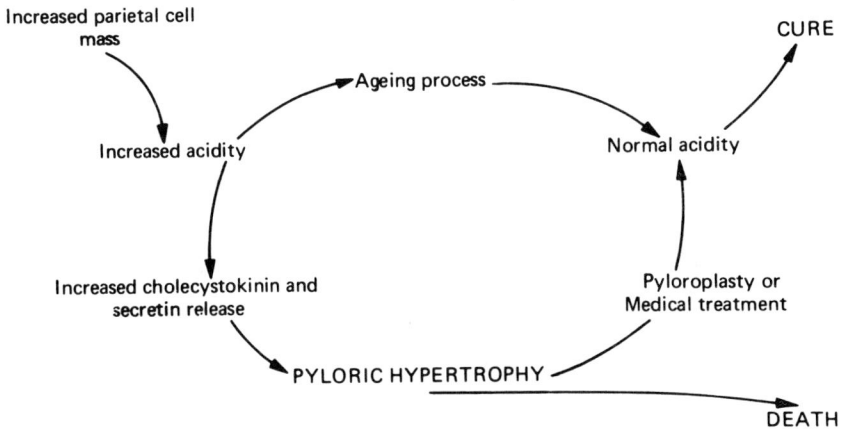

Increased parietal cell mass → Increased acidity → Increased cholecystokinin and secretin release → PYLORIC HYPERTROPHY → Pyloroplasty or Medical treatment → Normal acidity → CURE

Ageing process → Normal acidity

PYLORIC HYPERTROPHY → DEATH

Figure 3. Hypothetical model for production of infantile pyloric stenosis (From Rogers et al 1975, used by permission)

Clinical Features

Some of the conditions seen unduly frequently in association with pyloric stenosis are listed in Table IV. Although several are syndromes in which the infant is of low birth weight, the general tendency is for the disorder to be less common in pre-term infants and more frequent than expected in high-birth weight babies. (Czeizel, 1972). A surprisingly large proportion of patients (17.5%) have a history of vomiting frank blood, coffee-grounds or brown streaks, and this is presumably due to gastritis resulting from stasis, or to reflux oesophagitis. It does not itself mean that hiatus hernia must be considered, although the clinical association of the two conditions is well recognised. A rather puzzling complication sometimes seen in babies with pyloric stenosis is jaundice. The serum bilirubin in these infants is mostly unconjugated. The jaundice is not usually present from the neonatal period, but develops after a few weeks, either shortly before or after vomiting commences. It persists until the tumour is operated upon, after which it rapidly resolves. There is no

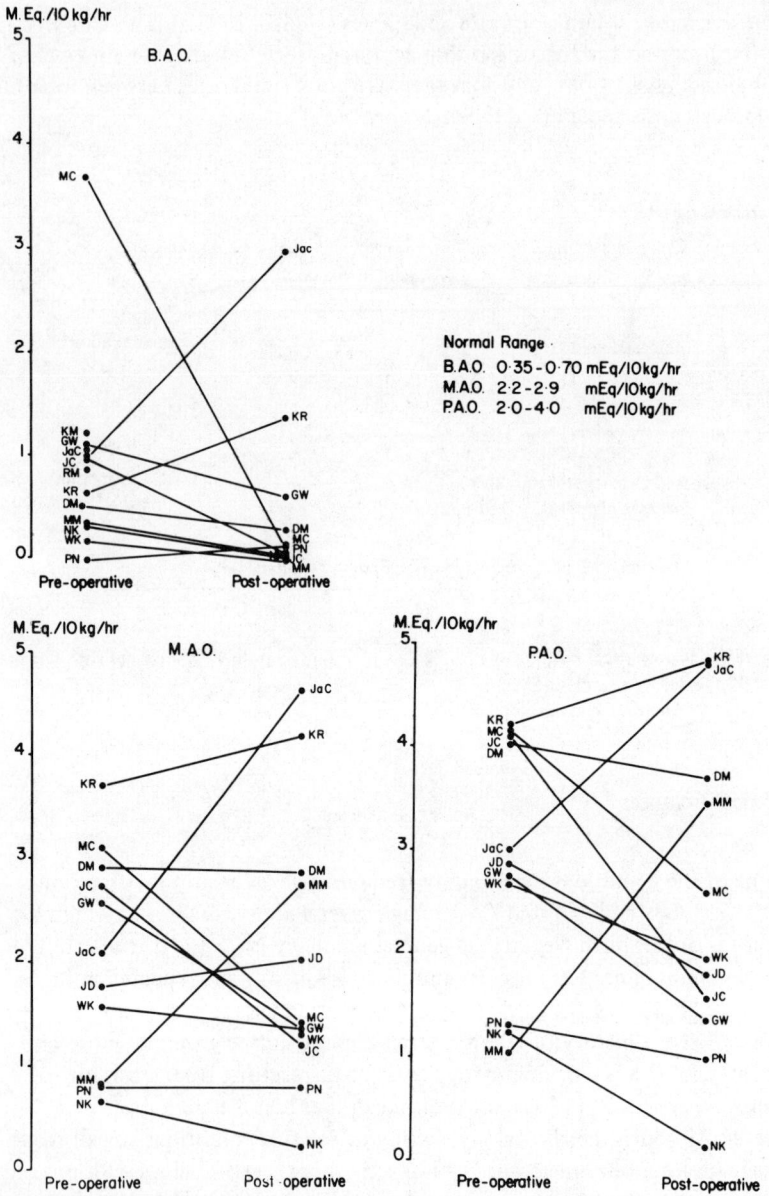

Figure 4. Basal, Maximal and Peak Acid Output in 11 infants before and 1 week after Ramstedt's operation

evidence that it is secondary to biliary obstruction. The most likely explanation is that the effects of gastric obstruction are similar to those of starvation, which is a standard way of inducing jaundice in patients with deficient hepatic glucuronyl transferase (Gilbert's disease). The incidence of jaundice in pyloric stenosis, about 3%, is very close to the estimated incidence of Gilbert's disease among blood donors (D Owens, 1974, personal communication).

TABLE IV. Infantile Hypertrophic Pyloric Stenosis: Associated Conditions

Oesophageal atresia and tracheo-oesophageal fistula
Partial thoracic stomach (Hiatus hernia)
Duodenal ulcer
Cystic Fibrosis
Phenylketonuria
Chromosome abnormalities:
  Trisomy 18
  XO Turner's syndrome
  Long Arm deletion 21
Smith-Lemli-Opitz syndrome
Amsterdam Dwarfs syndrome
Thalidomide embryopathy
Rubella embryopathy
Nocturnal enuresis
? Malignancies
Maternal myasthenia gravis

IDIOPATHIC INFANTILE VOMITING ('PYLOROSPASM')

Most infants with persistent vomiting have neither a hiatus hernia, nor a pyloric tumour. It is possible that they have some of the functional abnormalities of pyloric stenosis, but lack an adequate genetic endowment to express the full condition. This is suggested by the frequency with which sibs of infants with pyloric stenosis suffer from milder forms of vomiting. Controversy about the existence of 'pylorospasm' has raged almost since Hirschsprung's description of pyloric stenosis in 1888.

    Wood and Astley (1952) studied 22 infants with vomiting of uncertain origin. They found that there were two distinct groups: Persistent and Non-Persistent vomiters. The former have clinical features very similar to those of hiatus hernia and, subsequently, 4 of the 10 infants in this category proved to have a small loculus of thoracic stomach on repeated barium examination. Infants in this category usually improve when their feeds are thickened, but on average they continue to vomit until the 8th month of life. By contrast, the 12 Non-Persistent vomiters resembled babies with pyloric stenosis. Five of them were submitted to surgery but no tumours were found although atypical, ill-defined 'tumours' which were softer than usual had been palpated in all, as well as in a further 3 not operated upon. The radiological features in this group were suggestive of pylorospasm. The antrum was narrowed for periods of 10 minutes to 1 hour, but eventually relaxed. Peristalsis was seen in the narrow segment, which is not usual in true pyloric stenosis. The increased gastric peristalsis characteristic of pyloric stenosis is not seen in pylorospasm. Astley, describing the condition in 1975, believes that these radiological appearances may occur in a number of conditions causing vomiting in infancy, and emphasises the difficulty in distinguishing pylorospasm from true stenosis in some cases. Although such babies do not respond very well to therapeutic measures, the condition is self-limiting. The average age of onset was three weeks, and vomiting ceased at a mean of 10 weeks.

In a study of 771 vomiting babies, 273 were identified only because of the symptom being specially sought in a hospital nursery, and the remaining 498 had persistent vomiting with or without other major symptoms. In the latter group, 43 were diagnosed as 'pylorospasm', and their clinical features included forceful vomiting with mucus present in the ejected material, visible peristalsis, and a palpable contractile thickening (but not a distinct tumour) of the pylorus (Craig, 1961).

It is probable that in time this 'idiopathic' group will be eroded as we identify some specific causes. Cow's milk protein intolerance may be one of these, and hiatus hernia will be diagnosed more readily now that the radiological features have been more clearly defined. Functional pyloric hold-up appears to be related to gastrointestinal hormones, and it may be that developments in this field will help to explain this familiar syndrome.

References

Astley, R (1975) *Paediatric Gastroenterology.* (Ed) C M Anderson and V Burke. Blackwell, Oxford. Page 518
Becker, M, Fritsch, W P, Hausaman, T U and Rotthauwe, H W, (1975) *Meeting of European Society for Paediatric Gastroenterology, Brussels*
Benson, P F and King, M M R (1964) *Guy's Hospital Reports, 113,* 354
Carré, I J (1959) *Archives of Disease in Childhood, 34,* 344
Carré, I J (1975a) *Paediatric Gastroenterology.* (Ed) C M Anderson and V Burke. Blackwell, Oxford. Page 55
Carré, I J (1975b) *Idem,* Page 60
Carré, I J and Astley, R (1960) *Archives of Disease in Childhood, 35,* 484
Carter, C O and Evans, K A (1969) *Journal of Medical Genetics, 6,* 233
Chrispin, A R, and Friedland G W (1967) *Thorax, 22,* 422
Craig, W S (1961) *Archives of Disease in Childhood, 36,* 451
Czeizl, A (1972) *Idem, 47,* 978
Darling, D B, Fisher, J H and Gellis, S S (1974) *Pediatrics, 54,* 450
Dodge, J A (1970) *Nature, 225,* 284
Dodge, J A (1972) *Journal of Psychosomatic Research, 16,* 1
Dodge, J A (1971a) *MD Thesis, University of Wales.* Page 89
Dodge, J A (1971b) *Idem,* Pages 129–130

Dodge, J A (1973) *Clinics in Gastroenterology, 2,* 523
Friedland, G W, Dodds, W J, Sunshine, P and Zboralske, F F (1974) *American Journal of Roentgenology Radium Therapy and Nuclear Medicine, 120,* 305
Gellis, S S (1975) *Year Book of Pediatrics.* Page 196
Karim, A A (1975) *MCh Thesis, Queen's University of Belfast*
Karim, A A, Morison, J E and Parks, T G (1974) (abstract) *British Journal of Surgery, 61,* 327
Lari, J, and Lister, J (1972) *Archives of Disease in Childhood, 47,* 201
Lister, J and Wright, T (1967) *Proceedings of the Royal Society of Medicine, 60,* 449
Orellana, W, Darke, C S and Dodge, J A (1975) (To be published)
Pellerin, D, Bertin, P and Tovar, J A (1974) *Annales de Chirurgie Infantile, 15,* 7
Revill, S and Dodge, J A (1975) (abstract) *Archives of Disease in Childhood, 50,* 746
Rogers, I M, Davidson, D C, Lawrence, J, Ardill, J and Buchanan, K D (1974) *Archives of Disease in Childhood, 49,* 796
Rogers, I M, Drainer, I K, Moore, M R and Buchanan, K D (1975) *Archives of Disease in Childhood, 50,* 467
Roviralta, E (1950) *Archives Francaise des Maladies de l'Appareil Digestif, 39,* 1103
Toyama, W M (1969) *American Journal of Surgery, 117,* 650
Wood, B S B, and Astley, R (1952) *Archives of Disease in Childhood, 27,* 562

Discussion

DR WILSON   You mentioned sitting the baby upright and thickening of feeds in the treatment of this condition. Have you used 'Gaviscon'?

DODGE   Yes, but only in a few babies. It seems to be quite helpful, but I have not done a proper study. Gaviscon forms a foam on the surface of the gastric contents, and if it is regurgitated it is antacid and should protect the oesophagus.

DR PROSSER   What about carob seed flours, or metoclopramide (Maxolon)?

DODGE   In true hiatus hernias carob flours are much less effective than posture. Studies have shown that sitting the baby up is far better than thickening the feed, whereas thickening the feed alone is quite useful in babies with idiopathic vomiting without hiatus hernia. As far as I know, there has not been a proper study of metoclopramide, but in the two babies we have tried it on it seems to be very effective. One infant who had a partial thoracic stomach, who for some unknown reason rapidly deteriorated at the age of about 15 months, had a Ramstedt's operation instead of a fundoplication of the stomach and he was completely cured of symptoms. I think the correlation between pyloric dysfunction and problems at the hiatus is a very important one involving a lot of things including circulating gastrin.

DR LITTLEWOOD   I would support that infant Gaviscon has a dramatic effect on the regurgitating infant, but I suspect in the one with the partial thoracic stomach, it is going to be like Nestargel and not be nearly so effective.

95

DR MELLOR   I would like to ask if we have any information about head growth and posture if it is continued during a large part of the first six months of life.

DODGE   The head certainly gets flat. As time goes on this wears off and in fact it is not a gross malformation at any stage but if you look at a whole group of these babies they do have rather flattened heads.

The Neonatal Hepatitis Syndrome

A P MOWAT

Conjugated hyperbilirubinaemia in infants is never benign and always demands investigation. The majority of infants will have a variety of what we call the neonatal hepatitis syndrome. This may be defined as an inflammatory disease of the liver with conjugated hyperbilirubinaemia, biochemical and pathological evidence of hepatocellular necrosis with inflammatory cell infiltrate in the portal tracts and hepatic parenchyma. This definition should not imply that the cause is infectious. It might well be metabolic. There are many synonyms for this syndrome such as bile retention syndrome of infancy, intrahepatic cholestasis, and obstructive cholangiopathy of infants. The pathology of this condition is very variable. A distinct feature commonly seen is multinucleated large hepatocytes but this does not occur in all cases; it tells nothing of the aetiology, prognosis, nor of associated structural abnormalities. These multi-nucleated giant cells may occur in hepatitis or in biliary tract lesions. There are many causes or classifications of this syndrome (Sass-Kortsak, 1974) such as idiopathic hepatitis, biliary atresia, hepatitis of known infectious cause or due to inherited metabolic disorders, sepsis, intrahepatic cholestasis, and less frequent causes such as erythroblastosis, choledochal cyst, and gallstones. Infections associated with prolonged obstructive jaundice are given in Table I. The most important are septicaemia and urinary tract infections. Listeria, syphilis and toxoplasmosis are important since there are agents for treating these infections. The others are of academic interest only, since no therapy is available. Of the metabolic causes the most important are galactosaemia and fructosaemia since specific dietary therapy is so effective.

TABLE I. Infectious Causes of Hepatitis Syndrome in Infancy

Cytomegalovirus	Bacterial sepsis
Rubella virus	*Treponema pallidum*
Hepatitis B virus	*Toxoplasma gondii*
Herpes simplex	Listeria
Coxsackie B virus	
Varicella virus	
Zoster virus	

These conditions are easily diagnosed if the urine is tested for non-glucose reducing substances, but it is vital to test the urine when the patient is receiving the offending monosaccharide. Galactosaemic patients particularly, are liable to septicaemia and often require intravenous glucose influsion on admission. It is often at this time that it is remembered to test the urine which unfortunately may then be free from galactose, and the diagnosis may be missed or not made until irreversible hepatic or central nervous system damage has occurred. In some instances a very careful dietary history is essential before fructosaemia may be suspected. A specific diagnosis of tyrosinosis requires determination of serum and urinary amino acids but the diagnosis may be suspected if the Phenistix test is positive in urine. This condition, too, may occasionally respond to specific dietary treatment.

Cystic fibrosis and Niemann-Pick disease are infrequently complicated by hepatitis. Alpha-1 antitrypsin deficiency is the metabolic abnormality most frequently associated with the neonatal hepatitis syndrome in the UK.

With all these conditions to be considered, the clinician requires a fairly comprehensive scheme of investigation to identify the specific causes of the neonatal hepatitis syndrome as well as to try to determine whether there is a surgically correctable abnormality such as a choledochal cyst in the biliary tree. Investigations should include urine analysis, haematological studies, blood group determination, prothrombin time, liver function tests, X-ray of long bones for evidence of generalised intrauterine infection, upper gastrointestinal tract series, ultrasound examination of the abdomen, sweat electrolytes, alpha-1 antitrypsin phenotyping, ECG, as well as examination of urine and stools for bilirubin content.

In an epidemiological study in South East England, we found that the incidence of the neonatal hepatitis syndrome was approximately 1 in 2000 live births with an equal incidence of hepatitis associated with deficiency of the serum protein alpha-1 antitrypsin and extrahepatic biliary atresia (Cottrall et al, 1974). An indication of the relative frequency of the various causes and structural lesions associated with neonatal hepatitis syndrome is given in Table II. Alpha-1 antitrypsin deficiency is thus the major recognised cause of neonatal hepatitis. The remainder of this paper will deal with two conditions, neonatal hepatitis syndrome associated with alpha-antitrypsin deficiency and extrahepatic biliary atresia.

Alpha-1 antitrypsin is a serum glycoprotein normally present in a concentration of about 200 mg/100 ml but it increases in infections, pregnancy and with drugs, including oral contraceptive agents.

Disease is associated with severe genetically determined deficiency and takes two forms: hepatitis beginning in the newborn period and progressing to cirrhosis with death in early adult life, or emphysema starting early in adult life. Not all subjects develop these illnesses and rarely the two may co-exist together. These disease states are both associated with a serum concentration of around 40–60 mg/100 ml and with a slow migrating alpha-1 antitrypsin if we examine the serum alpha-1 antitrypsin in an acid starch gel electrophoretic system. Using this technique, many alleles of alpha-1 antitrypsin may be separated. They are designated alphabetically by their electrophoretic mobility. The most commonly found allele is M and such individuals are designated PiM (protease inhibitor). Disease is only commonly associated with the slow moving PiZ phenotype but Pi Nil in which there is virtually no serum alpha-1 antitrypsin, has also been associated with the disease (Cook, 1974).

TABLE II. Neonatal Hepatitis Syndrome — King's College Hospital Study 1970—74

CLASSIFICATION BY AETIOLOGY & STRUCTURAL ABNORMALITY

Extrahepatic biliary atresia		32
Choledochal cyst		2
Neonatal hepatitis of known cause		32
Alpha-1 antitrypsin deficiency	24	
Galactosaemia	1	
Tyrosinosis	1	
Hepatitis B virus infection	2	
Rubella	2	
Toxoplasmosis	1	
Rhesus isoimmunisation	1	
Idiopathic hepatitis		71

The biochemical explanation for the predisposition to disease associated with PiZ phenotype is not known, but the alpha-1 antitrypsin in such individuals lacks one of the four carbohydrate side chains which are normally present on alpha-1 antitrypsin. As yet there is no biochemical explanation for the different phenotypes (Sharpe, 1975).

Liver biopsy from patients with hepatitis complicating alpha-1 antitrypsin deficiency shows features of hepatitis with cholestasis. There is a variable inflammatory cell infiltrate, particularly in the portal tract and often increased fibrous tissue. Commonly seen are discrete, magenta coloured diastase resistant PAS positive globules which are seen in hepatocytes throughout the liver but often maximal in the periportal zones. These appear to be specific for alpha-1 antitrypsin deficiency. They are not found, however, before 12 weeks of age (Talbot & Mowat, 1975).

Just what predisposes these infants to hepatitis is not clear. Recent studies by Svegar suggest that only 10—20% of PiZZ infants develop significant liver disease. Although we had earlier suggested that hepatitis B antigen was a frequent predisposing factor, subsequent studies have not confirmed this observation (Porter et al, 1972). Aagenaes (Aagenaes et al, 1964) has proposed that an intrauterine insult causing low birth weight may be important, but some of the infants we have studied have had normal birthweights (Table III). The age of onset and duration of jaundice in some of over 30 patients we have studied is given in Table IV. In general, the more severe hepatitis in terms of the serum bilirubin concentration, and duration of jaundice, the worse the prognosis, but this is not universally true. I have seen one child who had a mild jaundice lasting only 10 days, but who had by three months of age a well marked cirrhosis and developed persistent ascites by 11 months.

TABLE III. PiZZ Infants with Liver Disease
Birthweight compared with appropriate weight for gestational age (as %)

%	Male	Female	TOTAL
< 5	4	2	6
5−10	0	0	0
11−25	4	1	5
26−50	4	2	6
51−75	0	2	2
76−95	0	0	0
> 95	0	2	2
	12	9	21

TABLE IV. Jaundice in Patients with Hepatitis and Alpha-1 Antitrypsin Deficiency

| Age of Onset | | Duration | |
Days	Number	Weeks	Number
< 5	9	4	2
5−14	6	4−8	2
15−28	6	9−12	6
35	1	13−16	3
56	1	17−20	2
		> 20	4
	23		19

Although the patient rapidly recovers from the hyperbilirubinaemia, serum alkaline phosphatase and aspartate aminotransferase levels rarely return to normal and most of these children go on with a chronic hepatitis and may be gradually developing cirrhosis although they are clinically well.

The serious nature of hepatitis associated with alpha-1 antitrypsin is reflected in Table V, which gives the data at the age stated on a total of 30 patients with liver disease associated with alpha-1 antitrypsin deficiency. The five who died all died from complications of cirrhosis. Many have clinical abnormalities; those who were clinically normal had biochemical abnormalities where tests were done, and the four children who are recorded as being clinically well, had no recent liver function tests.

100

TABLE V. *Current Clinical Status of Infants with PiZZ Phenotype and Liver Disease in Infancy*

Age at last follow-up	Dead	Clinically Abnormal	Clinically Normal	Biochemical Abnormality
1 yr	1	6	0	1
1–2 yrs	2	1	1	1
2–3 yrs			1	1
3–4 yrs	1	1		2
4–5 yrs			1	2
5–6 yrs				
6–7 yrs		2		
6–8 yrs			1	
13–14 yrs	1			

In hepatitis associated with alpha-antitrypsin deficiency we define a group of children who generally have a severe hepatitis which will in many instances progress to cirrhosis in childhood or early adult life. There are however, reported a few instances of adults aged between 20 and 30 who have had a hepatitis syndrome and are now clinically well with normal liver function tests and only mild increase in portal fibrosis, (Sass-Kortsak, 1974) but such a favourable outcome seems exceptional.

EXTRAHEPATIC BILIARY ATRESIA

There is now good evidence for believing that in many instances extrahepatic biliary atresia is an acquired condition. It is by far the most serious cause of obstructive jaundice in infancy; only about 5% of cases have a distal obstruction with dilated proximal, bile-containing, bile ducts which allow drainage by standard surgical procedures. Although a number of long-term survivors have been reported following operations on such children (Berenson et al, 1974), many of the 5% of patients who are operable do go on to develop cirrhosis and its complications. For most children and their parents extrahepatic biliary atresia is a grim illness, usually leading to death by two years of age. The operation of hepatic portoenterostomy developed in Japan by Kasai some 15 years ago has given new hope for such patients with reports of survivors to the age of 17 years being reported (Kasai, 1974). Recent literature from the Japanese group suggests that when the diagnosis has been made by 70 days of age, they have been able to obtain bile drainage in 7 out of the 8 infants with total obliteration of the extrahepatic bile ducts and no dilated proximal ducts or indeed macroscopically patent bile ducts. This data is now being confirmed from other centres (Lilley, 1975). Thus the frequency of potentially surgically remediable lesions in the biliary tract is much higher than seemed likely a few years ago when only choledochal cysts and the rare cases referred to above were considered correctable. In many infants with acholic stools in whom no cause for hepatitis can be established, the clinician therefore has a great responsibility to establish diagnosis of biliary atresia. It is also necessary that we make this diagnosis as early as possible.

Clinical features on standard liver function tests do not distinguish patients with extrahepatic biliary atresia from those with severe cholestasis and intact extrahepatic ducts. Infants with extrahepatic biliary atresia usually have a normal birthweight and in the first 1–3 months of life gain weight and grow satisfactorily despite their jaundice and do not have the gross features of cirrhosis and its complications we are familiar with in late cases. The diagnosis can only be confirmed by examination of the bile ducts but we would wish to avoid laparotomy in patients with hepatitis and intact ducts. The observation of Thaler and Gellis (1968), that laparotomy and careful examination of the extrahepatic biliary system caused an increased incidence of cirrhosis, is often challenged, particularly by surgeons, but has never been refuted. Although it is arguable that with current surgical, anaesthetic and radiological techniques these conclusions may no longer be valid, it is difficult to envisage that laparotomy can ever be a benign investigation particularly in hepatitis. Humanitarian and economic considerations must also cause us to avoid laparotomy if we can do so without jeopardising the patient's welfare. Unfortunately, indirect methods of diagnosing extrahepatic biliary atresia, such as the ratio of serum bile salts, the red cell haemolysis test and alpha fetoprotein which have been claimed to be of diagnostic value, have either been refuted or not confirmed in practice.

We find two investigations helpful; percutaneous liver biopsy under local anaesthetic, and the [131]I Rose Bengal faecal excretion test. In extrahepatic biliary atresia we will find widened portal tracts with prominent distorted, elongated angulated bile ducts, increased periportal fibrosis and inflammatory cell infiltrate, and preservation of normal cell architecture. There will be considerable cholestasis. In hepatitis there is prominent hepatocellular necrosis with disorganisation of liver cell cords and much giant cell transformation. There is inflammatory cell infiltrate in the portal tracts and in the parenchyma. Cholestasis is also prominent, particularly within hepatocytes. There will be focal bile duct proliferation but the severity of the bile duct lesion is much less than that of the hepatocellular lesion. There is unfortunately no single histological feature which is characteristic of either biliary atresia or hepatitis.

Nevertheless, we have found this investigation of considerable discriminatory value. In 80 infants who were subsequently considered to have intact extrahepatic bile ducts, the biopsy was correctly interpreted as hepatitis in 74, but in 6 biliary atresia could not be excluded. In the patients who had atresia, and had biopsies done before 12 weeks of age, the incidence of correct diagnosis was lower. Of 20 biopsies, 6 were considered definite biliary atresias, 9 were probable, but in 5 hepatitis seemed the most likely diagnosis. For this reason, we routinely perform an [131]I Rose Bengal faecal excretion test in infants with acholic stools.

It is important that the stools be collected uncontaminated with urine. An excretion of < 10% indicates insignificant bile flow compatible with atresia or severe cholestasis. If the biopsy is diagnostic of biliary atresia, we advise immediate laparotomy. Otherwise we give oral cholestyramine in a dose of 1g four times a day and continue this while we repeat the Rose Bengal excretion test 18—21 days later. In atresia, the excretion does not rise above 10% with this measure (Campbell et al, 1974). In hepatitis the excretion is likely to rise above 10% but unfortunately this does not happen in every case. For example, the one patient we have identified as having intrahepatic biliary hypoplasia with intact extrahepatic duct excreted only 7% on repeated testing. Thus by using these two investigations in parallel we can avoid laparotomy in all but a very few patients with hepatitis and intact extrahepatic ducts and have not overlooked any cases of extrahepatic biliary atresia.

If the observations made by Kasai and co-workers apply to infants with extrahepatic biliary atresia outwith Japan, it becomes vital that we try to make the diagnosis of extrahepatic biliary atresia before the age of 70 days. This will require that cases are referred to centres with appropriate diagnostic facilities at an early stage. This has not been happening hitherto; for example, of the 34 patients with extrahepatic biliary atresia we have studied, only 8 were operated on before 70 days of age. Only 4 of these had hepatic portoenterostomy, none were successful. Two of the patients operated on at around 5 months of age, had a hepatic portoenterostomy performed and developed bile drainage. Unfortunately, both of these children although still alive 18 months and 2 years later, do have recurrent attacks of ascending cholangitis and indubitably are developing cirrhosis. Ascending cholangitis is still a major complication following hepatic portoenterostomy although modification in the surgical anastomosis appear to have diminished the frequency of this. A further hazard of advising early surgery in suspected extrahepatic biliary atresia is that this might cause an increased number of infants with intrahepatic lesions and intact extrahepatic ducts to be submitted to laparotomy with the risks of possible destruction of their normal, patent but collapsed hypoplastic ducts by indiscreet surgery.

MEDICAL MANAGEMENT

Patients with the neonatal hepatitis syndrome often have retention of bile salts. High tissue concentrations of these are perhaps damaging to the liver and also to other tissues. A distressing consequence is pruritus. Cholestyramine in a dose of between 6 and 16 g/day given in the form of Questran will reduce serum bile salts levels and ameliorate or control the pruritus. In addition, serum lipid levels decrease and xanthomata may disappear. Side effects from this seem to be infrequent. A second major problem is fat malabsorption due to diminished or absent bile flow and the effect of lack of bile salts on fat digestion and absorption. This leads to calorie malnutrition and deficiencies of fat soluble vitamins. These effects may be mitigated by substituting medium-chain triglycerides for ordinary fat in the milk or in the diet. Fat soluble vitamins must be given in doses of between 2 and 4 times recommended daily allowances, occasionally parenterally. Serum calcium, phosphorus, prothrombin time should be monitored. When ascites complicates cirrhosis, it may often be controlled for some months with thiazides and spironolactone given with potassium supplements. Parents of patients with extrahepatic biliary atresia greatly appreciate what we can do to prevent unnecessary suffering by close attention to details in management. Paediatricians have a responsibility to provide such support.

References

Aagenaes, O, Fagerhol, M, Elgejo, K, Munthe, E, and Hovig, T (1964) *Postgraduate Medical Journal, 50,* 365
Berenson, M M, Gard, A E, Moody, F G (1974) *Gastroenterology, 66,* 266
Campbell, D P, Poley, J R, Alaupovic, P and Smith, E I (1974) *Journal of Paediatric Surgery, 9,* 699
Cottrall, K, Cook, P J L and Mowat, A P (1974) *Postgraduate Medical Journal, 50,* 376
Cook, P J L (1974) *Postgraduate Medical Journal, 50,* 362
Kasai, M (1974) *Progress in Paediatric Surgery, 6,* 5
Lilley, J R (1975) *Paediatrics, 55,* 12
Porter, C A, Mowat, A P, Cook, P J L, Haines, D W G, Sshilkin, K B and Williams, R (1972) *British Medical Journal, 3,* 435
Sass-Kortsak, A (1974) *Paediatric Clinics of North America, 21,* 777
Sharpe, O (1975) *Paper Presented at International Meeting on Paediatric Liver Disease, Paris.* (In Press)
Talbot, I C and Mowat, A P (1975) *Journal of Clinical Pathology, 28,* 559
Thaler, M M and Gellis, S S (1968) *American Journal of Diseases in Children, 116,* 257

Discussion

MR FREEMAN   As a surgeon, I would agree with a lot of what Dr Mowat says. It is interesting that in a lot of biliary atresias, they pass black meconium and this is very strong evidence in favour of an acquired lesion. The second thing I would like to say is that I find it hard to accept the evidence that surgery is an inhumane procedure for these babies in these days of anaesthesia, and that it does any harm. I think that laparotomy and operative cholangiography should just be at the bottom of the list of investigations, when it is done by 70 days post-delivery. Thirdly, I would say I have been doing the Kasai procedure for about six or seven years and although I was quite excited initially I have become a little bit disillusioned.

There is a very good editorial by Koop from Philadelphia in a recent 'Journal of Paediatric Surgery', trying to put sense into this rather confused picture.

104

He thinks we should rename this condition 'Progressive Biliary Disease after Birth', and that probably the intrahepatic atresia is just part of a spectrum of hypoplasia and non-drainage of the bile ducts. Presumably some vascular accident, or something else, happens to these extra hepatic ducts and causes the atresia. The most important thing, though, is that I do not think you can tell, except by looking at the extra hepatic duct system, and injecting, whether or not there is a lumen present. He goes on to show that the Kasai operation is a very unphysiological procedure because you dissect out the whole porta hepatis, and you take out the fibrous chunk of tissue which really represents the confluence of the left and right hepatic ducts, and join your jejunum on to this. Now if you take that tissue and section it, and if you can find lumina in there of 200 ml or more in size, those patients will have a chance to drain bile. If you section that tissue and there is *no* duct present, no operation in the world will work. In successful Kasai operations, if you look at the tissue you take out it will give you the prognosis as to whether the operation is likely to work or not. There will still be a group of hypoplastic ducts and completely atresic ducts and an intervening group with minute little ducts, but these are the only ones in which a surgeon can help.

MOWAT I think there is very little I can add. I just wanted to say that a lot of the children with extra hepatic atresia also have intra hepatic atresia as well and even in some cases where you find the bile duct you can still have problems.

QUESTION FROM AUDIENCE Some people have reported the value of alpha-feto protein in distinguishing between neonatal hepatitis and hepatic biliary atresia. Could we have Dr Mowat's comments?

MOWAT Dr Johnson and Dr Kohn of Roehampton took samples from some of our patients and so far they have examined something like 60 infants. They found in *some* of the hepatitis patients high levels which were quite different from the extra-hepatic biliary atresia patients but most had absolutely similar levels.

QUESTIONER So it is not likely to be a very useful test?

MOWAT No.

QUESTION FROM AUDIENCE It has been claimed that extra hepatic biliary atresia is due to a defective secretion of bile, that in fact the bile ducts are suffering from disuse atrophy. Would it not be a good idea to promote the secretion of bile with cholestyramine, or corticosteroids perhaps, before contemplating laparotomy? Could we have Dr Mowat's experience of the treatment of the children in whom surgery was not feasible, when they were treated with cholestyramine?

MOWAT   Well the problem with giving drugs like cholestyramine is that it may in certain circumstances increase bile flow, but it is so difficult to measure bile flows that I do not have any data. I think that biliary hypoplasia because of the lack of bile production is one of the things that really terrifies me in encouraging people towards early laparotomy, because if we have inexperienced surgeons, they may well cut away all the extra hepatic biliary apparatus, although all we really need to do is wait until the bile starts coming.

DR McNEISH   I would like to make a plea to those like Dr Mowat who see a lot of these cases, because I think there have been very few papers in the literature which have been so influential as the one paper of Thaler and Gellis (1968) saying that it is a dangerous thing to do a laparotomy. I would think there *was* a place, not, as you point out for the inexperienced surgeon, but for a surgeon who, like yourself, sees many, to repeat this work, and to be rather bold and do a laparotomy, and then tell us perhaps in a couple of years' time what happens. I would predict you will not find that Gellis was correct.

MOWAT   Well, one just does not have the opportunity to do that. I disagree with Mr Freeman that it is a humanitarian thing to do a laparotomy if you can avoid it. I think it is unjustified to do a laparotomy if you do not have to.

QUESTION FROM AUDIENCE   There are a number of procedures which have been published, to try and differentiate extra hepatic atresia from intra hepatic atresia, measuring serum bile acids. Most of these papers are dogged by the fact that in most centres there are very small numbers of these patients. One of the problems I find is not knowing what the natural history of neonatal hepatitis syndrome is. How active should we be in trying to correct the obstructive jaundice that we do see? Should we use steroid therapy, should we use cholestyramine treatment, or not? Just what is the natural history of this condition?

MOWAT   You have asked a lot of questions. As far as the published criteria for hepatitis and intra hepatic and extra hepatic biliary atresia, we have checked all the problems, techniques and theories and found they have not held up. We have not checked lipoprotein X.

McNEISH   We had one patient in Birmingham where lipoprotein X was absent and yet this child had atresia.

MOWAT   Well, that is disheartening, because we have checked 7 or 8 for lipoprotein X, and it seemed to be useful. As to the natural history of the disease, I really cannot give you an answer to that, but certainly the alpha-1-antitrypsin deficient ones are a severe problem. We have nothing specific to offer them. I think one has to look very hard for sepsis, galactosaemia, fructosaemia. My feelings are that the idiopathic variety will come out to have a pretty good prognosis. Of our idiopathic ones, I think we have something like 7 with cirrhosis, the others seem to be pretty well. We have not identified any feature in the newborn period which picks out the ones who will get cirrhosis.

References

Koop, C E (1975) *Journal of Paediatric Surgery, 10,* 169

Diarrhoea

Intestinal Infection

J T HARRIES

Intestinal infection is a major health problem throughout the world, and carries an appreciable mortality and morbidity; this is particularly the case during infancy and in those developing parts of the world where malnutrition is common. This paper briefly reviews some of the more important aspects of intestinal infection in childhood. For more detailed accounts on bacterial and viral enteritis, the reader is referred to forthcoming reviews by Harries (1976) and Tripp and Harries (1976); for parasitic infection the reader is referred to Ebrahim (1976).

BACTERIA

Incidence and Pathogenic Species

The reported incidence of 'pathogenic' bacteria cultured from the stools of children with acute diarrhoea has varied from 4 to 33 per cent over the last 20 years, the commonest species being 'enteropathogenic' strains of *E. coli,* Salmonella and Shigella. In recent years it has become clear that enterotoxin-producing strains of *E. coli,* with somatic serotypes not recognised as 'enteropathogenic', can cause diarrhoea; these strains cannot be identified by conventional laboratory techniques and require techniques such as ligated rabbit loops or tissue culture. The term 'enteropathogenic' therefore requires redefinition, and the aetiological importance of bacteria in gastrointestinal infection in children is probably much greater than previous reports have indicated.

Pathophysiological Mechanisms

Enteropathogens can be classified as invasive (Shigella, Salmonella, and some strains of *E. coli*) or non-invasive (*V. cholera* and *E. coli*) according to their capacity to penetrate bowel mucosa. Invasive species predominantly affect the ileum and colon to produce dysentery (stools containing blood, pus and mucus), whereas the non-invasive organisms affect the small intestine and result in watery diarrhoea.

There is now compelling evidence that the heat-labile enterotoxins elaborated by *V. cholera* and *E. coli* induce small intestinal secretion by activation of the mucosal enzyme adenyl cyclase and the generation of high concentrations of cyclic AMP (Kimberg, 1974).

VIRUSES
(see Lancet, 1975)

There is no good evidence that enteroviruses or adenoviruses can result in intestinal disease. Viruses described as 'rotaviruses' or 'duoviruses' have, in recent years, been detected in the stools of children with acute gastroenteritis from several parts of the world. Although not yet unequivocally proven, it is probable that these viruses are aetiological agents in an appreciable proportion of young children developing acute gastroenteritis. There is evidence that these viruses and the Norwalk agent produce morphological abnormalities of the small intestinal mucosa, but there is no evidence that gastric mucosal structure is altered (Widerlite et al, 1975).'Viral enteritis' may therefore be a more appropriate description of the disease, rather than gastroenteritis; similarly when bacteria are implicated, 'bacterial enteritis' may be a preferable term. The pathophysiological mechanisms responsible for viral-induced gastrointestinal disease are not known.

PARASITES

TABLE I. Intestinal Parasites

* PROTOZOA
Amoebiasis
Giardiasis
Coccidiosis
* HELMINTHS
Hookworms
Ascariasis
Strongyloidiasis
Trichuriasis
Taeniasis
Cysticercosis
Ecchinococcosis
Diphyllobothriasis
Schistosomiasis

The more important intestinal parasites that are known to infest man may be broadly classified as protozoa and helminths (Table I). All these are reviewed in detail elsewhere (Knight et al, 1973; Ebrahim, 1976), and only giardiasis will be

111

considered in this section. *Giardia lamblia* is a flagellate protozoon which has both a trophozoic and cystic stage; it inhabits the duodenum and jejunum and is one of the most common parasites of man. Diarrhoea may be acute and of short duration, or may be prolonged and lead to failure to thrive. In adults with hypogammaglobulinaemia Ament and Rubin (1972) have shown patchy mucosal abnormalities in the small gut which improved following eradication of the parasite. Improvement in mucosal abnormalities associated with giardiasis following eradication of the protozoon in the absence of a recognisable immunodeficiency state has only recently been convincingly demonstrated (D. Ogilvie & J. T. Harries, unpublished observations). We investigated a 7 year old boy with Down's syndrome who had a history of failure to thrive and loose, bulky stools. Intestinal biopsy showed severe partial villous atrophy, and giardia were identified in duodenal juice and the biopsy specimen; tests of humoral and cell-mediated immunity were normal. Eradication of the parasite resulted in a return of mucosal morphology to normal and clinical improvement. Diagnosis rests on identification of the parasite in stools or duodenal juice; the absence of parasites in stools by no means excludes their presence in the proximal small gut.

DISEASE DETERMINANTS

TABLE II. Disease Determinants of Intestinal Infection

---

* THE EXTERNAL ENVIRONMENT

Health Services Safe water supplies
       Sewage disposal
       Solid waste disposal
       Development of welfare clinics
Improved management and follow up of infective enteritis and malnutrition
Health and nutrition education of the public
Economic and agricultural measures
Breast feeding.

* INTERACTIONS BETWEEN HOST AND BACTERIA

Gastric juice
Small gut motility
Resident flora
Immune systems

Gastrointestinal infection results from a complicated series of interactions between the external environment, the pathogen and the host and its resident bacterial flora (Table II); colonisation of the bowel by sufficient numbers of bacteria results in disease. Knowledge of many of these interactions is minimal, and further work in this area is of great importance to the future control of infective enteritis. In the developing countries factors in the external environment

112

such as improvement in health services, development of infant welfare clinics, improved management and follow up of enteritis and malnutrition, health and nutrition education to the public, and economic and agricultural measures deserve high priority. Breast feeding protects against infection, and its present decline throughout the world may be accompanied by an increased frequency of enteric infection.

Gastric juice, small gut motility, the resident flora, and immune systems all play a role in maintaining the normal ecology of the gut, and provide defence mechanisms against pathogen invasion.

COMPLICATIONS

The two most important complications of acute enteric infection are hypernatraemic dehydration (i.e. serum sodium > 150 mM/l), and the development of a protracted diarrhoeal syndrome (i.e. more than 4 watery stools per day for longer than 2 weeks). Permanent neurological sequelae may occur in up to 16 per cent of infants with hypernatraemic dehydration, and peripheral gangrene, renal vein thrombosis and medullary necrosis may also be complications. Protracted diarrhoea may persist for several weeks or months and lead to severe nutritional disturbances. The pathophysiological mechanisms responsible for this syndrome are not clear, but sugar and/or cow's milk protein intolerance are of importance in some patients.

MANAGEMENT

Acute Disease

The single most important factor in management of acute enteritis is the correction of fluid and electrolyte imbalance. As in cholera, the oral administration of glucose-containing solutions in heat-labile enterotoxin *E. coli* disease may prove to be an important first-aid measure. Although there is general agreement that the correction of hypernatraemia should be gradual (i.e. over 36–72 hours), opinion on the composition of the intravenously administered solutions is controversial. Persistent oliguria or anuria may reflect renal failure, and may be an indication for peritoneal dialysis.

Protracted Diarrhoea

Elimination of dietary sugars and/or cows' milk protein is effective in a proportion of patients. Dietary manipulations may be unsuccessful and, in these circumstances, intravenous feeding may be life-saving. In those infants who respond to dietary treatment, reintroduction of a normal diet is usually possible after 2 to 3 months.

References

Ament, M E and Rubin, C E (1972) *Gastroenterology, 62,* 216

Ebrahim, G J (1976) In *Essentials of Paediatric Gastroenterology.* (Ed) J T Harries. Churchill Livingstone, London (to be published). Chapter 12

Harries, J T (1976) *Essentials of Paediatric Gastroenterology.* (Ed.) J T Harries. Churchill Livingstone, London (to be published)

Kimberg, D V (1974) *Gastroenterology, 67,* 1023

Knight, R, Schultz, M G, Hoskins, D W and Marsden, P D (1973) *Gut, 14,* 145

Lancet (1975) 'Rotaviruses of man and animals,' *i,* 257

Tripp, J H and Harries, J T (1976) In *Essentials of Paediatric Gastroenterology.* (Ed) J T Harries. Churchill Livingstone, London (to be published). Chapter 10

Widerlite, L, Trier, J S, Blacklow, N R and Schreiber, D S (1975) *Gastroenterology, 68,* 425

Bile Salts and Diarrhoea

K W HEATON

The laxative properties of bile salts* have been known for centuries and have been exploited in many nostrums. It is still possible to prescribe and to buy in the chemist's shop proprietary laxatives containing bile salts. Only in the last few years, however, has this property of bile salts been studied and its clinical significance revealed. Some early workers in this field (Forth et al, 1966) made the interesting suggestion that in healthy subjects excessive dehydration of the stool, hence constipation, are prevented by the small amount of bile salt which normally enters the colon. Certainly, constipation is a side effect of treatment with resins which bind and inactivate bile salts in the colon. Certainly too, any disease or therapeutic procedure which markedly increases the flux of bile salts into the colon causes diarrhoea. The most obvious example is oral chenodeoxycholate therapy for the dissolution of cholesterol-rich gallstones. Diarrhoea (or relief of constipation) is the main side effect, though it is seldom troublesome when the dose is 1 g/d. This dose roughly doubles the normal input of bile salts into the colon, which is about 500 mg/d.

The Role of the Colon in Normal Bile Salt Physiology

As an absorptive organ, the colon is not essential in bile salt economy. Patients with ileostomies do not excrete excessive quantities of bile salts unless the terminal ileum has been resected as well (Percy-Robb et al, 1971). However, the bacterial flora of the colon plays an important role in modifying bile salts chemically. The two main changes undergone by bile salts in the colon are deconjugation and 7-α-dehydroxylation. Deconjugation, which also occurs in the terminal ileum, is the hydrolysis of the peptide bond which links a bile acid to its glycine or taurine sidechain. The resulting free or unconjugated bile acids — cholic, chenodeoxycholic and deoxycholic — are to some extent reabsorbed. The efficiency of this reabsorption is very high in the ileum, thanks to its active transport system, but probably only 30—40% in the colon where the only mechanism

---

* In this paper, the terms bile salt and bile acid are used interchangeably. For a discussion of this and other aspects of bile salt terminology, the reader is referred to Heaton (1972).

available for bile acid absorption is passive diffusion. Unabsorbed bile acids in the colon are subject to removal of the 7-α-hydroxyl group. By this means anaerobic bacteria, especially Bacteroides, convert cholic into deoxycholic acid and chenodeoxycholic into lithocholic acid. Lithocholic acid is very insoluble and only trace amounts are absorbed. Deoxycholic is quite well absorbed and after conjugation in the liver it functions as a normal bile salt. The circulating bile acid pool consists therefore of about 45% cholic acid (trihydroxy), 35% chenodeoxycholic and 20% deoxycholic (both dihydroxy), all three being conjugated with glycine and taurine in a ratio of about 3:1.

In normal human faeces the main bile salts are deoxycholate and lithocholate. The concentration of deoxycholate in faecal water is about 4 mmoles/1. This is within the range of concentrations at which dihydroxy bile acids influence colonic function.

Effects of Bile Acids on Colonic Function

It was shown many years ago that bile enemas cause prompt defaecation in dogs, and more recently that bile acids infused into the rabbit caecum at 2—4 mmol/l concentrations increase colonic motor activity (Kirwan et al, 1974). This suggests that bile salts may cause diarrhoea by accelerating colonic transit. However, cholegenic diarrhoea is usually ascribed to the actions of bile salts on colonic absorption, the main features of which were established in a classic study by Forth et al (1966). Absorption of water from tied off loops of rat colon was completely blocked by unconjugated deoxycholic acid (DC) in the low concentration of 1 mmol/1. Unconjugated chenodeoxycholic acid (CDC) was also very potent. Indeed, the threshold concentration for inhibition of absorption by CDC was only 0.4 mmol/1, whereas the concentration in normal colonic contents was up to 4 mmol/1. Compared with these dihydroxy bile acids, the trihydroxy acid cholic acid was less effective, and conjugates of all three were ineffective.

The relevance of these findings to man was established by Mekhjian, Phillips and Hofmann (1971) in an exhaustive (and one suspects, exhausting) series of experiments on 20 healthy volunteers. Test solutions were perfused via a long per-oral tube into the caecum and the effluent collected from the rectum for analysis of water and electrolyte movement. When the test solution contained DC 3 mmol/1 or CDC 5 mmol/1 there was not merely inhibition of water absorption, but actually net secretion of water or rather of an isotonic sodium chloride solution. Unconjugated cholic acid had no effect even at 10 mmol/1. Conjugation with glycine and taurine seemed to make no difference to the secretory effects of the dihydroxy bile acids. These findings differ somewhat from the rat data of Forth et al (1966) but have been confirmed in the dog (Mekhjian & Phillips, 1970). In the dog the colon was also observed to secrete excess mucus.

Thus, dihydroxy bile acids in physiological or near-physiological concentrations increase colonic motility, decrease absorption, stimulate secretion and possibly induce mucus production.

116

Effects of Bile Acids on Small Intestinal Function

Dysfunction of the small intestine can of course cause diarrhoea, presumably because the volume of ileal effluent exceeds the absorptive capacity of the colon (normally about 1500 ml/day; Phillips & Giller, 1973). It is of interest therefore that, experimentally, bile acids have powerful effects on the small intestine. Indeed, with in vitro incubation, DC and CDC, and to a lesser extent cholate, inhibit all the metabolic processes of the small intestinal mucosa, including active transport of sugars and amino acids and various synthetic processes (Dietschy, 1967). There may even be structural damage to the villi (Low-Beer et al, 1970). However, these non-specific cytotoxic actions are largely an artefact of in vitro preparations, in which bile acids accumulate in the mucosa. In vivo, such actions can be demonstrated but only at much higher bile salt concentrations (Teem & Phillips, 1972). Nevertheless, bile salts do affect small intestinal function at physiological concentrations. In human volunteers, perfusion of the jejunum with 2.5 or 3 mM conjugated DC and CDC inhibited water and electrolyte absorption and at higher concentrations evoked secretion of an isotonic fluid (Wingate et al, 1973; Russell et al, 1973). However, Wingate et al made the important observation that addition of lecithin to the perfusion fluid abolished these effects. Lecithin and similar polar lipids (such as monoglyceride) are always to be found in the jejunum during digestion, that is during the periods when bile salts are present in the small bowel. This implies that, even in vivo, the effects of pure bile acid solutions on the jejunum may be an artefact of the laboratory. On the other hand, the ileum is likely to be exposed to bile salts without the protective polar lipids being present, since lipids are largely or wholly absorbed in the jejunum, whereas bile salts remain in the intestine until they reach the terminal ileum. Judged by in vitro experiments, the ileum seems to be more sensitive than the jejunum to the absorption-inhibiting effects of bile acids (Wingate, 1973; Caspary, 1974). However, this is probably because ileal mucosa avidly takes up bile acids from the bathing fluid whereas jejunal mucosa can only acquire them by passive diffusion. Therefore intracellular concentrations are likely to be higher with ileal preparations. In vivo, bile salts are unlikely to accumulate in the ileal mucosa since it is constantly perfused with blood which carries away absorbed materials. In fact, in vivo perfusion studies suggest that the ileum is *less* sensitive to bile salts than the jejunum. Thus, Harries and Sladen (1972) found that 1 mM DC inhibited water absorption in the rat jejunum but over 5 mM DC was required to have the same effect in the ileum. In man, perfusion of the ileum with 2.5 mM CDC or DC, or with 5 mM GCDC or GDC inhibited water and electrolyte absorption and even caused some net secretion (Krag & Phillips, 1973).

Sugar absorption by the jejunum is inhibited by in vivo exposure to pure DC solutions (Gracey et al, 1971) although the concentration may have to be as high as 5 mM (Harries & Sladen, 1972). In man glucose absorption is slightly inhibited by glycine conjugated bile acids, but only when lecithin is absent from the perfusing solution (Wingate et al, 1973).

How relevant are these experimental findings to human disease? In particular, does contamination of the small bowel by faecal bacteria able to deconjugate bile salts result in impaired small bowel function? In other words, is the diarrhoea and malabsorption of the stagnant loop syndrome due, at least in part, to the toxic effects of unconjugated dihydroxy bile acids on the small bowel mucosa? This hypothesis has been debated for 15 years, and is still unproven. However, evidence in its favour is accumulating. Using rats with surgically created self-filling blind loops, Gracey et al (1971) showed impaired ability of the small bowel mucosa to transport monosaccharide sugars in the vicinity of the blind loops. This impairment correlated with the density of anaerobic flora and with the extent of bile salt deconjugation. The small bowel mucosa of patients with the stagnant loop syndrome has not been studied in this way. However, it has been shown to be morphologically abnormal, especially on electron microscopy (Ament et al, 1972). The damaged microvilli and other changes could be caused by DC or CDC, but other bacterial products could also be responsible. The steatorrhoea of the stagnant loop syndrome is usually blamed on low concentrations of conjugated bile salts, resulting from bacterial deconjugation (Tabaqchali & Booth, 1970). However, this too could be due to toxic damage to the jejunal mucosa (Ament et al, 1972).

Mechanism of Bile Acid Induced Changes in Intestinal Function

Recently there has been much interest in how bile acids alter intestinal function. The simplest explanation is that their detergent properties damage mucosal cells. This would fit with the greater toxic effects of the dihydroxy bile acids, since these are the better detergents. With liver cell preparations it has been possible to reproduce bile acid toxicity with a synthetic detergent Triton-X-100 (Denk et al, 1971). Of more direct relevance, Saunders et al (1975) have shown that an anionic detergent which is prescribed as a laxative (dioctyl sodium sulphosuccinate, DSS) inhibits water absorption in the colon of the rat, and in the small intestine of rat and man. At 1 mM concentration, which could be achieved clinically, DSS actually induced net water secretion in the human jejunum. The parallel with the natural detergents, bile salts, is clear.

Binder and his colleages at Yale have adopted a different approach. Their hypothesis is that bile salts induce the colonic mucosa to secrete by increasing the intracellular concentration of cyclic AMP. This would resemble the action of cholera toxin on small bowel mucosa; the toxin is believed to increase intestinal adenylate cyclase, the enzyme which catalyses the production of cAMP. In favour of this hypothesis, Binder et al (1975) have shown that the level of cyclic AMP in the mucosa of the rat colon increased by 54% when it was exposed for 3 hours to 6 mM taurochenodeoxycholic acid. At the same time, the potential difference and short circuit current across the mucosa increased, which implies increased sodium transport, consistent with increased cyclic AMP activity.

118

Finally they showed that treating the mucosa with cyclic AMP itself increases short circuit current and alters sodium transport in exactly the same way as the bile acid. The only gaps in the argument have been neatly plugged by Conley et al (1975), who have shown that the concentration of adenylate cyclase in the rabbit colon increases markedly when it is exposed to deoxycholic acid. Furthermore, secretion of water increased 10-fold when the colon was treated with either 6 mM DC or dibutyryl cyclic AMP.

Disorders where Bile Acids Cause Diarrhoea — the Cholegenic Diarrhoeas

The experiments discussed above suggest that diarrhoea should occur whenever there is malabsorption of bile salts, hence increased entry of bile salts into the colon, and perhaps also whenever there is excessive bile salt deconjugation in the small intestine. Clinical experience suggests that this is in general the case.

Terminal ileal disease or resection is the model situation. The main site of bile salt reabsorption is the terminal ileum, and when the last 40 to 100 cm of the small intestine are resected there is usually troublesome watery diarrhoea. The diarrhoea is generally precipitated by meals and worst after breakfast. It often causes anal soreness or itching. Daily excretion of bile acids is increased 2- to 10-fold over the normal 300 to 500 mg/d. On analysis, faecal bile acids are found to have escaped dehydroxylation, and to consist mainly of cholic and chenodeoxycholic acids, instead of the normal deoxy- and lithocholic (Hofmann, 1972; Mitchell & Eastwood, 1972). This failure of microbial degradation may be due to rapid transit time through the colon, but it could also be due to inhibition of the colonic flora by the high concentrations of bile acids. Certainly, anaerobic bacteria are inhibited in vitro by unconjugated bile acids (Floch et al, 1971).

The best evidence that this bile acid flux or cholerrhoea is responsible for the diarrhoea is the dramatic relief obtained with cholestyramine therapy. In a dose of 4 grams with each meal, there is significant reduction in faecal weight and frequency (Hofmann & Poley, 1969). Faecal fat increases but not enough to have nutritional significance. With long-term treatment there is a small but definite risk of deficiency of fat-soluble vitamins, which should be countered by prescribing vitamins D and K. In practice, many patients can be managed satisfactorily with codeine phosphate.

The diarrhoea is considerably worse if the ileocaecal valve and ascending colon are resected as well as the terminal ileum (Cummings et al, 1973). The reason for this is not clear. It may simply be that the right colon is normally the main site of water absorption. As an additional factor, the ileo-caecal sphincter probably delays the passage of small bowel contents into the colon and so allows more time for bile salt absorption in the remaining ileum.

Even with minor ileal resections, there is usually some steatorrhoea. The reason for this is that with interruption of the enterohepatic circulation there is a defici-

119

ency of bile salts available to be secreted into the duodenum. This is often described as a reduction in the bile salt pool. However, it is more accurate to say that there is no bile salt pool. The term pool implies miscibility and exchangeability between old and newly synthesised material. If there is no circulation there can be no mixing or exchange. The bile salts accumulated in the gallbladder during fasting are mostly or wholly newly synthesised. They will be used only once instead of the normal 20 times. They are all that is available for the digestion of the next meal. After a prolonged fast, for example overnight, the liver (which is synthesing bile salts at maximal rate since the normal feedback inhibition by recycled material has been lost) may be able to accumulate 2 g of bile salts in the gall-bladder, which is near the $2\frac{1}{2}$ to 3 g size of the normal circulating pool (Abaurre et al, 1969). However, between later meals there is much less time for new synthesis and so for the later meals less stored bile salt is available in the gallbladder. When the concentration of bile salts in the duodenum during digestion is measured, it is found to be only slightly subnormal after breakfast but very low after later meals, e.g. 1–2 mM instead of the normal 4–12 mM (van Deest et al, 1968). At these low concentrations there are insufficient bile salt micelles to solubilise the products of fat digestion, some of which therefore escape absorption. (For a fuller discussion of the interrupted enterohepatic circulation, see Dowling, 1972; Heaton, 1972; and Hofmann, 1972.)

Steatorrhoea itself can cause diarrhoea. With extensive ileal resections (>100 cm) steatorrhoea is severe, probably because of the shortened time and place available for fat absorption on top of bile salt deficiency. Diarrhoea is relieved little if at all by cholestyramine but responds to restriction of dietary fat intake, or to replacement of the normally preponderant long chain triglycerides by medium chain triglyceride, whose absorption does not require micellar solubilisation (Hofmann & Poley, 1969, 1972). Long chain fatty acids are themselves cathartic and have been shown by perfusion studies to inhibit water and electrolyte absorption in the human colon (Ammon & Phillips, 1973). Patients with ileal resection or bypass may therefore suffer from fatty acid diarrhoea as well as bile acid diarrhoea, depending on the amount of ileum lost.

Extensive ileal mucosal damage of any cause can lead to cholegenic diarrhoea (or fatty acid diarrhoea). The main cause is certainly Crohn's disease, but occasionally it follows radiation ileitis and malignant infiltrations.

Postvagotomy diarrhoea has long been an enigma, but recent evidence points to bile acid malabsorption as an important cause, at least in the small minority who have persistent watery stools. In 1973, Allan et al reported that the mean faecal bile acid excretion in seven such patients was 2100 mg/d, compared with 688 mg/d in normal controls. The same group have gone on to show in a controlled trial that this diarrhoea is relieved by cholestyramine (R I Russell, personal communication, 1975), which confirms the experience of Ayulo (1972) and of Condon et al (1975). Why patients who have undergone vagotomy and a drainage procedure should have difficulty in reabsorbing their bile acids is at present quite obscure. Further investigations of ileal function in these patients will be of interest. Meanwhile, the possibility of small bowel bacterial over-growth must be considered since even in vagotomy patients without diarrhoea there is evidence of increased bacterial degradation of bile salts (Arnesjö & Ståhl, 1974). However, if it occurs, this bacterial overgrowth must be limited to the ileum, since the jejunum is not colonised particularly often in vagotomy patients who develop diarrhoea (Browning et al, 1974).

Cystic fibrosis poses a similar problem. Weber and his colleagues (1973) measured the faecal bile acids of 24 children with pancreatic insufficiency secondary to cystic fibrosis and found it to be 743 mg/d, which is much higher than in age-matched controls (110 mg/d) and not significantly different from infants with ileal resection. The most obvious explanation of these findings is malabsorption of bile acids, and this has been confirmed by reports that the half-life of isotopically labelled bile acids is abnormally short in cystic fibrosis (Weber et al, 1975; Watkins et al, 1975). Bile acid loss was proportional to faecal fat excretion, and improved when pancreatic replacement therapy was given (Weber et al, 1973). On the other hand, children with steatorrhoea due to coeliac disease did not have cholerrhoea. This led to the suggestion that bile acid absorption is inhibited by large quantities of unhydrolysed fat, or other undigested nutrients in the ileum. This situation would have a precedent in that vitamin B_{12} malabsorption sometimes occurs in pancreatic insufficiency and can be corrected by treatment with pancreatic extracts (Bernstein & Herbert, 1973).

Two facts complicate this interpretation. Firstly, bile acid flux has not been reported in adults with pancreatic failure. Indeed, breath tests suggest it does not occur (Sherr et al, 1971; James et al, 1973). Secondly, coeliac disease may be inappropriate as a control situation in which there is simple malabsorption: There is now evidence that in coeliac disease the ileal mucosa develops supernormal absorptive capacity, as a compensatory phenomenon for the subnormal jejunal function (Silk et al, 1975). This could give the coeliac patient a supernormal capacity for bile acid absorption, which is a specialised function of ileal mucosa. By this means, coeliac patients could maintain normal faecal bile acids, although in other circumstances malabsorption and steatorrhoea wash bile acids into the colon.

This raises the question — can diarrhoea itself cause bile acid malabsorption by rushing bile salt molecules past the active transport sites in the terminal ileum? The only published studies bearing on this question are those of Meihoff and Kern (1968). They induced watery diarrhoea in four volunteers by giving them large volumes of 10% mannitol to drink. The rate of excretion of radioactive cholic acid was doubled, but this was a trivial change compared with that observed in six patients with ileal resection. It hardly merited the term bile acid malabsorption.

121

Small bowel contamination.   The possibility has already been discussed that small bowel dysfunction in the stagnant loop syndrome is caused by the toxic action of deconjugated bile acids. The evidence must still be regarded as inconclusive. Some protagonists of the idea have suggested that chronic diarrhoea in infants with sugar malabsorption is the result of bacterial contamination of the small intestine (Gracey et al, 1969), the implication being that deconjugated bile acids cause sugar malabsorption by impairing the ability of the mucosa to hydrolyse disaccharides (Gracey et al, 1975) or to transport monosaccharides (Gracey et al, 1971). However, when Challacombe et al (1974) tested this hypothesis they found deconjugated bile salts in the duodenum of only one out of seven infants with chronic diarrhoea (three of whom had secondary sugar intolerance). The situation may be different in tropical countries, where even healthy subjects harbour a considerable bacterial population in the upper small intestine. In a study of malnourished Guatamalan children it was found that those with diarrhoea had not only increased bacterial contamination but also deconjugated bile acids in their duodenal fluid in a mean concentration of 3 mM (Schneider & Viteri, 1974). However, much more evidence is necessary before it can be accepted that chronic unexplained diarrhoea in general is caused by bacteria let alone mediated by deconjugated bile acids.

Other diarrhoeal conditions   The pathogenesis of *diabetic diarrhoea* is obscure. Recently, Condon et al (1975) have reported that cholestyramine treatment completely relieved four patients with intractable diabetic diarrhoea. This obviously suggests that the diarrhoea was cholegenic in origin, and further reports on this condition will be awaited with interest. In a double-blind study in Boston, longstanding diarrhoea attributed to the *irritable colon syndrome* was relieved by cholestyramine therapy in five out of twelve patients (Schapiro et al, 1970); surprisingly, no confirmatory reports have appeared. Relief with cholestyramine has also been reported in a single patient with *watery diarrhoea and acquired hypogammaglobulinaemia* (Gleich & Hofmann, 1971). Excessive bile salt losses in the faeces have been reported in two cases of severe *idiopathic infantile diarrhoea* present since birth, but diffuse ileal disease had not been excluded (Balistreri et al, 1974).

Tests for Cholegenic Diarrhoea

The only direct test of whether a patient's diarrhoea is due to excess bile acids in the colon is a therapeutic trial of cholestyramine. Other bile acid-sequestrants may also be effective but have not been evaluated. When cholestyramine is given in a dose of 4 g (e.g. one sachet of Questran) with each meal, there should be an immediate reduction in the fluidity and frequency of the stools.

There are a number of tests for bile acid malabsorption, which for practical purposes is the sole cause of cholegenic diarrhoea. The glycocholate breath test is much the simplest, but it is the least specific as it merely detects abnormal bacterial breakdown of bile salts, and so is also positive in the stagnant loop syndrome. A liquid test meal containing $5-10\ \mu Ci$ of ^{14}C-glycocholate is given to the patient, and expired air is analysed hourly for the radioactivity in CO_2. The only special apparatus required is a liquid scintillation counter. Occasional patients with ileal disorders and diarrhoea give a negative response. Further details are given in the papers by Fromm and Hofmann (1971), Sherr et al (1971) and James et al (1973).

More specific but much more complicated tests for bile acid malabsorption are the chemical assay of faecal bile acids, measurement of faecal radioactivity after taking a radioactive bile acid by mouth, and analysis of biliary radioactivity after labelling the bile salt pool with a radioactive bile acid. Bile acids labelled with stable isotopes are also available. Details of these techniques, which are of research interest only, are given by Hofmann et al (1970). Detection of a high glycine/taurine conjugation ratio in the bile has been advocated as a relatively simple screening test for bile acid malabsorption (Bruusgaard & Hess Thaysen, 1970), but its specificity has not been established and it involves duodenal intubation to obtain a sample of bile.

SUMMARY

Bile salts are cathartics, and can cause diarrhoea if they are given by mouth or if they enter the colon in excessive quantities due to failure of reabsorption in the terminal ileum. Dihydroxy bile salts are potent inhibitors of colonic water and electrolyte absorption and in near-physiological concentrations they can induce colonic mucosa actually to secrete fluid. Bile salts can also stimulate colonic motility. They act on colonic mucosa probably by inducing it to synthesise more cyclic AMP. Experimentally, dihydroxy bile salts act in a similar way upon small bowel mucosa but the physiological relevance of these findings is uncertain, and neither the diarrhoea nor the steatorrhoea of the stagnant loop syndrome can yet be confidently attributed to deconjugated bile salts. Resection of the terminal ileum, if extensive, will cause fatty acid rather than bile acid (cholegenic) diarrhoea. Non-ileal disorders believed to cause cholegenic diarrhoea include truncal vagotomy with drainage, cystic fibrosis and possibly diabetes. The best test for cholegenic diarrhoea is a therapeutic response to the bile salt-sequestering resin cholestyramine, and the use of this agent is the most effective treatment. The ^{14}C-glycocholate breath test is a simple and useful screening test.

References

Abaurre, R, Gordon, S G, Mann, J G and Kern, F (1969) *Gastroenterology, 57*, 679

Allan, J G, Gerskowitch, V P and Russell, R I (1973) *Gut, 14*, 423 (abstract)

Ament, M E, Shimoda, S S, Saunders, D R and Rubin, C E (1972) *Gastroenterology, 63*, 728

Ammon, H V and Phillips, S F (1973) *Gastroenterology, 65*, 744

Arnesjö, B and Ståhl, E (1974) *Scandinavian Journal of Gastroenterology, 9*, 601

Ayulo, J A (1972) *American Journal of Gastroenterology, 57*, 207

Balistreri, W F, Partin, J C and Schubert, W K (1974) *Gastroenterology, 66*, 832 (abstract)

Bernstein, L and Herbert, V (1973) *American Journal of Clinical Nutrition, 26*, 340

Binder, H J, Filburn, C and Volpe, B T (1975) *Gastroenterology, 68*, 503

Browning, G G, Buchan, K A and Mackay, C (1974) *Gut, 15*, 644

Bruusgaard, A and Thaysen, E H (1970) *Acta Medica Scandinavica, 188*, 547

Caspary, W F (1974) *European Journal of Clinical Investigation, 4*, 17

Challacombe, D N, Richardson, J M and Edkins, S (1974) *Acta Paediatrica Scandinavica, 63*, 581

Condon, J R, Robinson, V, Suleman, M I, Fan, V S and McKeown, MD (1975) *British Journal of Surgery, 62*, 309

Conley, D R, Coyne, M J, Chung, A, Bonorris, G G and Schoenfield, L F (1975) *Gastroenterology, 68*, 877 (abstract)

Cummings, J H, James, W P T and Wiggins, H S (1973) *Lancet, i*, 344

Denk, H, Greim, H and Hutterer, F (1971) *Gastroenterology, 60*, 187 (abstract)

Dietschy, J M (1967) *Federation Proceedings, 26*, 1589

Dowling, R H (1972) *Gastroenterology, 62*, 122

Floch, M H, Gershengoren, W, Elliott, S and Spiro, H M (1971) *Gastroenterology, 61*, 228

Forth, W, Rummel, W and Glasner, H (1966) *Archiv für experimentelle Pathologie und Pharmakologie, 254*, 364

Fromm, H and Hofmann, A F (1971) *Lancet, ii*, 621

Gleich, G J and Hofmann, A F (1971) *Americal Journal of Medicine, 51*, 281

Gracey, M, Burke, V and Anderson, C M (1969) *Lancet, ii*, 384

Gracey, M, Burke, V and Oshin, A (1971) *Scandinavian Journal of Gastroenterology, 6*, 273

Gracey, M, Burke, V, Oshin, A, Barker, J and Glasgow, E F (1971) *Gut, 12*, 683

Gracey, M, Houghton, M and Thomas, J (1975) *Gut, 16*, 53

Harries, J T and Sladen, G E (1972) *Gut, 13*, 596

Heaton, K W (1972) *Bile Salts in Health and Disease.* Churchill Livingstone, Edinburgh

Hofmann, A F (1972) *Archives of Internal Medicine, 130*, 597

Hofmann, A F and Poley, J R (1969) *New England Journal of Medicine, 281*, 397

Hofmann, A F and Poley, J R (1972) *Gastroenterology, 62*, 918

Hofmann, A F, Schoenfield, L J, Kottke, B A and Poley, J R (1970) In *Methods in Medical Research, Vol. 12.* (Ed.) R E Olson: Year Book Medical Publishers, Chicago, page 149

James, O F W, Agnew, J E and Bouchier, I A D (1973) *British Medical Journal, 3*, 191

Kirwan, W O, Smith, A N, Mitchell, W D and Eastwood, M A (1974) *Gut, 15*, 828 (abstract)

Krag, E and Phillips, S F (1973) *Journal of Laboratory and Clinical Medicine, 83*, 947

Low-Beer, T S, Schneider, R E and Dobbins, W O (1970) *Gut, 11*, 486

Meihoff, W E and Kern, F (1968) *Journal of Clinical Investigation, 47*, 261

Mekhjian, H S and Phillips, S F (1970) *Gastroenterology, 59*, 120

Mekhjian, H S, Phillips, S F and Hofmann, A F (1971) *Journal of Clinical Investigation, 50*, 1569

Mitchell, W D and Eastwood, M A (1972) *Scandinavian Journal of Gastroenterology, 7*, 29

Percy-Robb, I W, Jalan, K N, McManus, J P A and Sircus, W (1971) *Clinical Science and Molecular Medicine, 41*, 371

Phillips, S F and Giller, J (1973) *Journal of Laboratory and Clinical Medicine, 81*, 733

Russell, R I, Allan, J G, Gerskowitch, V P and Cochran, K M (1973) *Clinical Science and Molecular Medicine, 45*, 301

Saunders, D R, Sillery, J and Rachmilewitz, D (1975) *Gastroenterology, 68,* 980 (abstract)

Schapiro, R H, Heizer, W D, Goldfinger, S E and Aserkoff, B R (1970) *Gastroenterology, 58,* 993 (abstract)

Schneider, R E and Viteri, F E (1974) *American Journal of Clinical Nutrition, 27,* 788

Sherr, H P, Sasaki, Y, Newman, A, Banwell, J G, Wagner, H N and Hendrix, T R (1971) *New England Journal of Medicine, 285,* 656

Silk, D B A, Kumar, P J, Webb, J P W, Lane, A E, Clark, M L and Dawson, A M (1975) *Gut, 16,* 261

Tabaqchali, S and Booth, C C (1970) In *Modern Trends in Gastroenterology – 4.* (Ed.) W I Card and B Creamer. Butterworth, London, page 143

Teem, M V and Phillips, S F (1972) *Gastroenterology, 62,* 261

van Deest, B W, Fordtran, J S, Morawski, S G and Wilson, J D (1968) *Journal of Clinical Investigation, 47,* 1314

Watkins, J B, Tercyak, A M, Szczepanik, P and Klein, P D (1975) *Gastroenterology, 68,* 1087 (abstract)

Weber, A M, Roy, C C, Lepage, G, Chartrand, L and Lasalle, R (1975) *Gastroenterology, 68,* 1066 (abstract)

Weber, A M, Roy, C C, Morin, C L and Lasalle, R (1973) *New England Journal of Medicine, 289,* 1001

Wingate, D L (1973) *Gastroenterology, 64,* 824 (abstract)

Wingate, D L, Phillips, S F and Hofmann, A F (1973) *Journal of Clinical Investigation, 52,* 1230

Discussion

DODGE Dr Harries, do you think that in infective diarrhoea the problem starts by colonisation of the colon and works upward in a retrograde way, or do you think that bacteria are swallowed and first colonise the upper small intestine? A lot of the work that has been done was in animals, and in pigs in particular, which have a reservoir of bacteria in the stomach, which seem to spill over and go down into the small bowel; whereas I imagine, without any really good reason, that perhaps in humans it starts the other way and works up. This obviously has implications for bile salt deconjugation and so on.

HARRIES I think that the evidence with cholera at any rate suggests that this is colonisation downwards, but I think probably with *E. coli,* for instance, it may well be the other way around. Regarding your final point on bile salt conjugation, I think this is a controversial area in terms of its importance in infantile diarrhoea. Some interesting work came out of Gambia recently where they have intubated the duodenum of children with malnutrition, both with and without diarrhoea, and found very high counts of anaerobes (Heyworth & Brown, 1975).

There is another paper which has come from Guatemala, which has shown undoubted bile salt deconjugation (both tri- and di-hydroxy bile salts), in concentrations which would be expected to produce an inhibitory effect on absorption (Schneider & Viteri, 1974).

DR McNEISH If we talk of experimental data first of all, Williams Smith's experimental *E. coli* diarrhoea in pigs in which he colonised the gut — then the
pattern of colonisation is that these piglets have virtually no *E. coli* in their
oesophagus, nor indeed in the stomach, but as you cross from the stomach
into the duodenum some of the counts go up very rapidly and there is an
enormous growth of *E. coli* in the duodenum. He would only accept our
E. coli diarrhoea as a true infection if you have demonstrated that sort of system. Now most people have diagnosed *E. coli* diarrhoea in babies by looking
for certain serotypes in the stools, but we now think that *E. coli* which is truly
enteropathogenic is rather different. I think it fair to say that current studies
in Birmingham would support the Williams Smith hypothesis. In true acute
E. coli diarrhoea in infants, we have found the same situation as he did in his
experimentally colonised piglets, that is to say that there would be a rather
unspectacular upper intestinal flora, but we came upon the organisms in the
duodenum. Whether they have come from oral swallowing mechanisms, and
just a few of them cross the otherwise fairly hostile stomach but then multiply
in the duodenum, or whether they come from below, I do not think we know.
David Challacombe's work has been mentioned and he and others have shown
that in chronic diarrhoea you may get a generalised colonisation from mouth
to anus with high counts of faecal type organisms. One has to interpret the
duodenal counts in these babies with great caution, because they may well
have several organisms in high counts in their stomachs, in the oesophagus,
even in the throat swab. I am not saying that that means that they are not
affecting the duodenum, but that the *distribution* of organisms in chronic
diarrhoea seems to be rather different and this colonisation from one end to
the other seems to be a feature of chronic diarrhoea.

HEATON I always assumed that it was from the top down, but the point that
we need to remember is that the mouth has a very atypical flora, and I think
it is fair to say that all the organisms which you can get from the colon can
be isolated in the mouth, although obviously in infinitesimally smaller counts.
A patient with achlorhydria gets worse salmonellosis than those with normal
gastric acid, which gives importance to the idea of it coming from above. Now
as far as chronic diarrhoea and bile salt deconjugation are concerned, the paper
you mentioned from Guatemala I thought rather confusing and not very conclusive. The authors have undoubtedly shown concentrations up to 3 mmol
of free bile acids in the duodenal aspirates, but the odd thing is this is only in
those who recovered from protein-calorie malnutrition and yet continued to
have diarrhoea. It was not present while they still had malnutrition, and he
did not release any evidence, unfortunately, that antibiotic treatment affected
children's diarrhoea, which I thought was rather critical. I find this field of
chronic diarrhoea in infants and children and its relation to bacteria and the
correlation of bile salts in the upper bowel a very confused one.

DODGE Would you have any thoughts on the possible role of prostaglandins in producing diarrhoea? We have talked about adenyl cyclase in the cholera diarrhoea mechanism, but I wondered whether prostaglandins are involved because there is no doubt that prostaglandins can cause diarrhoea and that also they can activate adenyl cyclase.

HEATON As I understand it, the only disease in which they have definitely been shown to play a part, is in medullary carcinoma of the thyroid, a very rare condition. Whether they play a part in other diarrhoeas is anybody's guess.

McNEISH Just following on from that, it is quite interesting in a recent paper in 'Nature', in which they were investigating the effects of *E. coli* rather than cholera, they showed, as you might expect, that cyclic AMP production was stimulated through adenyl cyclase. They then went on to show that this system, which you would think might be exhausted, far from being so, was exquisitely sensitive to other stimulants of this pathway, including prostaglandins. They postulated that mechanism for the continuation of the diarrhoea, because we know, or believe we know, that in many cases of enterotoxic diarrhoea, the growth of organism may be over in perhaps two or three days and yet the symptoms may persist. They also postulated that once this system had been switched on, physiological amounts of other normal stimulants of the pathway would then have a greater than normal effect.

DR ROSEMARY EVANS Why do you have diarrhoea in immunodeficiency disorders?

HARRIES I find this very interesting and do not know the reasons, unless the patients have infection with *giardia lamblia* or other unusual pathogens.

DR JOHN MORRIS Would Dr Heaton comment on the fact that cholestyramine is not a harmless treatment in the long term, but may in fact induce severe bone changes, particularly in children?

HEATON We did record a patient who developed osteomalacia when she was on long term cholestyramine treatment for persistent diarrhoea. It was very effective in the treatment of diarrhoea but she developed osteomalacia. We cared for that easily enough of course, but there have not been any other reports of it. There has been a report on hypoprothrombinaemia, presumably indicating vitamin K deficiency and theoretically certainly one would expect gross malabsorption.

MORRIS Certainly in patients with chronic liver disease it can be very serious. In four patients with primary cirrhosis, cholestyramine precipitated fat-soluble vitamin deficiencies.

127

HARRIES   Dr Richard West in the Institute of Child Health, has been looking at absorptive function in children with hypercholesterolaemia treated with long term cholestyramine. Serum vitamin A and folate levels go down, as well as faecal fat, but I do not think anyone developed bone disease.

References

Heyworth, B and Brown, J (1975) *Archives of Diseases in Childhood, 50,* 27
Schneider, R E and Viteri, F E (1974) *American Journal of Clinical Nutrition, 27,* 788

128

Some Aspects of Sugar Intolerance

A S McNEISH

In the past decade, paediatricians have become very aware of the important clinical syndromes that may cause, or result from, dietary carbohydrate malabsorption. This paper is not meant to be comprehensive. I have chosen to discuss a few examples, mainly of secondary sugar intolerance, that illustrate important or controversial principles.

There are many recent reviews of the physiology of carbohydrate digestion and absorption from the intestine, and I particularly recommend the brief but up-to-date description by Gray (1975). The polysaccharides starch and glycogen, after hydrolysis by pancreatic alpha-amylase, yield 1,4-linked oligosaccharides of length 2 to 9 glucose units, and 1,6-linked alpha-limit dextrins with an average content of 8 glucose units. Further hydrolysis of these molecules is completed by the specific alpha-glucosidases that are embedded in the brush border membrane of the intestinal epithelial cell in a manner that leaves their active hydrolytic sites available at the brush-border surface. *Gluco-amylase* acts upon malto-oligosaccharides to produce glucose, and supplies 25% of total maltase activity. *Sucrase-isomaltase* (better called sucrase-alpha-dextrinase) can hydrolyse alpha-limit dextrins as well as maltose. This hybrid molecule represents 75% of total maltase activity. Sucrase of course also hydrolyses sucrose to glucose and fructose, and the remaining important dietary disaccharide lactose is hydrolysed by the betagalactosidase, lactase, to produce glucose and galactose.

Glucose (and galactose) at the brush border are transported into the call by the carrier-specific, Na$^+$- and energy-dependent mechanism first proposed by Crane (1965). The absorption of fructose is probably also by an independent specific carrier system.

It has recently been recognised that an 'unstirred layer' of intestinal contents overlies the luminal surface of the epithelial cell membrane (Winne, 1973). This layer, fractions of a millimetre thick, constitutes a diffusion barrier whose properties explain many of the discrepancies between kinetic studies of pure oligosaccharidases and in vivo experiments. The properties of this layer in various diseased states of infants are entirely unknown. Nevertheless it seems likely that fuller understanding of these properties would be rewarding.

It is not surprising that such complex mechanisms should be affected by

129

diseases involving the intestinal epithelium, leading to carbohydrate malabsorption with or without clinical evidence of intolerance.

It is important to distinguish between *sugar malabsorption,* which is diagnosed in essence by the interpretation of a variety of biochemical tests, and *sugar intolerance*, which term I think should be used to describe the abnormal clinical symptoms and signs that may result from ingestion of the offending sugar (Bayless et al, 1968). For example, as discussed later, lactose malabsorption is very common in untreated coeliac disease, yet it is seldom necessary to have to withdraw lactose from the diet of a coeliac child.

I consider the following to indicate or be associated with sugar malabsorption: a 'flat' blood glucose curve after an oral sugar load; increased short-chain organic acids or sugars in the faeces; lowered levels of intestinal disaccharidases. Sugar intolerance means failure to thrive, with abdominal distension, diarrhoea and vomiting after an oral sugar load, and with a prompt clinical response to an elimination diet. There are of course areas of overlap; for example infants with lactose intolerance will almost always have a flat blood glucose curve after lactose challenge, and decreased intestinal lactase. There are however exceptions even to this statement (see below, cows' milk protein intolerance), and the general distinction between malabsorption and intolerance needs to be remembered when interpreting the literature.

The congenital syndromes are well-known that result from deficiency of one specific enzyme concerned with the absorption of a particular sugar. The remainder of this paper concentrates on a few examples of sugar malabsorption, often multiple, whose causes or importance are less clear.

Sugar Intolerance in Coeliac Disease

The severe loss of intestinal villi that is the feature of untreated coeliac disease is inevitably accompanied by a loss of absorptive surface and a diminution of disaccharidase activities of the epithelial cells. 'Flat' lactose and glucose tolerance curves are common (Anderson, 1966) but the clinical importance of this malabsorption is less clear. Arthur et al (1966) believed that the majority of children with coeliac disease required a lactose-free diet in the early months of treatment. Some years ago, we found that all but 1 of 23 untreated coeliac children had lactose malabsorption, but only 1 of 23 (4%) required lactose withdrawal in order to control diarrhoea and allow weight gain (McNeish & Sweet, 1968). In that study, the finding of a stool pH of less than six correlated much better with true lactose intolerance than did the shape of the blood lactose curve after oral load.

It is obvious that the degree of lactose malabsorption will be influenced by the length of small intestine that is affected, while the presence or absence of watery acidic stools depends at least in part upon intestinal transit time and colonic absorptive function.

Sugar Intolerance Following Gut Surgery in Neonates

Burke and Anderson (1966) described a group of neonates who had sugar (particularly disaccharide) intolerance following gut surgery. In some, the symptoms could easily be explained by loss of small intestinal absorptive surface by surgical resection or by-pass, but in others the surgery involved only the large intestine (e.g. transverse colostomy for Hirschsprung's disease) and the cause of sugar malabsorption was less obvious.

In Birmingham, colleagues have recently found excess numbers and species of bacteria in the duodenal fluid of neonates who have recently had major gut surgery (Challacombe et al, 1974). There are several mechanisms, so far incompletely investigated, by which these organisms could influence sugar absorption. A direct luminal hydrolysis by the organisms; damage to intestinal epithelial cells; 'enterotoxic' alteration of fluid absorption or secretion; deconjugation of bile salts with resulting toxic depression of sugar transport (Gracey et al, 1969; Harries & Sladen, 1972); these possibilities need to be explored further.

In the meantime it is enough to be aware of the possibility that neonates who have had gut surgery may require dietary sugar restriction for several weeks.

The Role of Lactose Intolerance in Cows' Milk Protein Intolerance (CMPI)

Liu et al (1968) showed that the intestinal absorption of lactose was impaired when children who were recovering from CMPI were fed either whole milk or betalactoglobulin. Lubos et al (1967) studied a group of children with CMPI and observed that the maximum rise in blood glucose after an oral lactose load was in general reduced, but correlated rather poorly with intestinal lactase levels. Furthermore, features of frank lactose intolerance were uncommon. We have confirmed these observations, but their explanation remains unclear. It is possible that the lactose malabsorption in CMPI results from an interference with the transport of glucose and galactose into the epithelial cells, or is simply the result of loss of intestinal absorptive surface associated with a variable enteropathy. It should be noted in passing that Dr Wharton and colleagues (see elsewhere) have shown that, even in normal infants, there is a difference between the rate of lactose absorption from whole milk and the absorption rate from a simple lactose solution.

In summary, lactose malabsorption is common in CMPI but symptoms of frank intolerance are probably unusual.

Sugar Intolerance During, or Following, Acute Gastroenteritis

Some forms of acute gastroenteritis are associated with structural mucosal damage, and it is easy to understand how secondary disaccharide (and occasionally monosaccharide) intolerance can result. The possible effects of a soluble enterotoxin on carbohydrate absorption remain less well defined, and more studies are needed.

131

In practical clinical terms, it is the youngest infants, under six months, who are most likely to develop this type of secondary sugar intolerance, and any co-existing malnutrition is likely to aggravate matters further. The excellent studies of Torres-Pinedo and colleagues (see Rodriguez-de-Curet et al, 1970) and Lifshitz et al (1971) have taught us that lactose malabsorption is usually more important than either glucose or maltose malabsorption. There is known to be an increase in the numbers of duodenal bacteria in proportion to the degree of sugar malabsorption (Coello-Ramirez & Lifshitz, 1972) but whether this is an aetiological or a secondary feature requires further investigation.

Professor Charlotte Anderson (personal communication) has suggested that there is a case for giving a lactose-free formula for a few weeks to all infants under six months of age who develop gastroenteritis, because it is difficult to predict which infant will develop lactose intolerance. There is much to commend this approach.

Intractable Diarrhoea in Infancy

This incompletely understood syndrome is characterised by multiple digestive and absorptive abnormalities (Avery et al, 1968), and malabsorption of all disaccharides and monosaccharides is common. Reduction or alteration of oral carbohydrate intake is only a part of the complex dietary manipulation that is necessary, and intravenous elemental feeding may be required (Lloyd-Still et al, 1973). In our experience, disaccharidase deficiency may take months to resolve after successful nutritional resuscitation, and pancreatic function may also remain depressed for many weeks (R Nelson & A S McNeish, unpublished observations). During convalescence it is therefore prudent to reintroduce dietary carbohydrates singly and initially at low concentration.

Summary

Many infants with sugar intolerance are too ill to justify full initial investigation so that the preliminary diagnosis may have to be based on the response to dietary eliminations. A knowledge of the physiology of carbohydrate absorption is of vital importance in planning suitable diets and in interpreting the clinical course.

References

Anderson, C M (1966) *Archives of Disease in Childhood, 41,* 571

Arthur, A B, Clayton, B E, Cottom, D G, Seakins, J W T and Platt, J W (1966) *Lancet, i,* 172

Avery, G B, Villavicencio, O, Lilly, J R and Randolph, J G (1968) *Pediatrics, 41,* 712

Bayless, T M, Rosenweig, N S, Christopher, N and Huang, S-S (1968) *Gastroenterology, 54.* 475

Burke, V and Anderson, C M (1966) *Australian Paediatric Journal, 2,* 219

132

Challacombe, D N, Richardson, J M and Rowe, B (1974) *Archives of Disease in Childhood, 49,* 270

Coello-Ramirez, P and Lifshitz, F (1972) *Pediatrics, 49,* 233

Crane, R K (1965) *Federation Proceedings, 24,* 1000

Gracey, M, Burke, V and Anderson, C M (1969) *Lancet, ii,* 384

Gray, G M (1975) *New England Journal of Medicine, 292,* 1225

Harries, J T and Sladen, G E (1972) *Gut, 13,* 596

Lifshitz, F, Coello-Ramirez, P and Contreras-Gutierrez, M L (1971) *Journal of Pediatrics, 79,* 612

Liu, H-Y, Tsao, M U, Moore, B and Giday, Z (1968) *Gastroenterology, 54,* 27

Lloyd-Still, J D, Shwachman, H and Filler, R M (1973) *American Journal of Diseases of Children, 125,* 358

Lubos, M C, Gerrard, J W and Buchan, J W (1967) *Journal of Pediatrics, 70,* 325

McNeish, A S and Sweet, E M (1968) *Archives of Disease in Childhood, 43,* 433

Rodriguez-de-Curet, H, Lugo-de-Rivera, C and Torres-Pinedo, R (1970) *Gastroenterology, 59,* 396

Winne, D (1973) *Biochimica Biophysica Acta, 298,* 27

Cow's Milk Protein Intolerance

MARGOT SHINER, JANET BALLARD, C G D BROOK and S M D HERMAN

In an earlier paper on the effect of cow's milk on the small intestinal mucosa of infants allergic to proteins in the milk, we showed that challenge studies resulted in definite changes in mucosal immuno-pathology which in the early hours was suggestive of a local reaginic reaction. The infants described had clinical reactions to the milk challenge within two hours. Subsequently we have tested another four infants, suspected of milk allergy, in a similar manner. All of these showed no adverse clinical symptoms after one or more small doses of cow's milk over a period of 24 hours, yet in two of the four cases pronounced jejunal mucosal changes occurred. We now describe our investigation of these four infants to show that (1) intolerance to the proteins of cow's milk should be considered a definite disease entity, (2) clinical reactions to a milk challenge may be absent, and (3) jejunal biopsy before and after milk challenge is essential for diagnosis, especially in the absence of symptoms.

Patients

Four infants aged 5–11 months were investigated. All presented with failure to thrive and had diarrhoea and/or vomiting and patient 2 had intermittent blood in the stools. Patient 4 was the only one with a family history of allergy and he had mild eczema and sensitivity to ampicillin. Full investigations were carried out to exclude lactose intolerance, enteric infections and immune deficiency. When sensitivity to cow's milk was suspected the patients were taken off milk and put on either a soya bean formula or a hydrolysed casein formula. All made good progress on this regime. Patients 2 and 3 had previously been exposed to gluten.

After 3–12 weeks on the formulae the infants were admitted for challenge with whole cow's milk. We employed the following regime: (1) after a 12 hour fast, a baseline jejunal biopsy (O) was taken with the paediatric Crosby capsule. (2) blood was examined for haemoglobin, white cell count including eosinophils, immunoglobulins, serum complement (measured as β-1a), and the RAST test for IgE-specific antibodies to milk (Phadebas). This was followed by (3) administration by mouth of either a single dose of 30 ml of cow's milk and, in the

134

absence of symptoms, of several repeat doses over the next 8 hours up to a total of 150 ml; (4) after a further 12 hour fast the second jejunal biopsy was taken on the next day. This was immediately followed by repeat blood examinations. Both the biopsies and the blood tests were recorded in relation to the first milk challenge.

The mucosal biopsies were examined blindly by three different observers histologically, ultrastructurally and by immunofluorescence techniques.

Results

None of the four patients reacted clinically to the milk over the 24 hours following the start of the challenge.

Haematological data showed the following abnormal features: Patients 1, 2 and 3 were mildly anaemic, patients 1 and 4 had high initial serum IgE values (149 and 90 I.U./ml respectively) but patient 1 was the only one with circulating IgE-specific antibodies to milk (RAST test). The only changes observed in the serum after the milk challenge were an increase in β-1a which was observed in patient 1 at 4 hours and in patient 2 at 5 hours (84 and 90 mg% respectively). Normal levels were obtained after 18 and 23 hours respectively. It is particularly noteworthy that no eosinophilia was seen after the challenge in any of the infants, and that immune deficiency was not found.

Light microscopy (Table I)

The histology of the pre-challenge biopsies (O) showed a normal jejunal mucosa in patient 3 and a mild partial villous atrophy (N/PVA) in the other three patients. The histological appearances did not change in the post-challenge biopsies of patients 3 and 4, 12 and 22 hours respectively, after milk, whereas marked pathological appearances were noted in the post-challenge biopsies of patients 1 and 2 after 18 and 23 hours respectively. These consisted of shortening and broadening of villi, and intense inflammatory cell infiltration which included polymorphs (Figs. 1 and 2) and mast cells.

TABLE I. *Suspected cow's milk intolerance before and after milk challenge*

		Biopsies	Immunofluorescence of jejunal mucosa							
			IgG		IgM		IgA		IgE	C3
Pt. No.	Age in Months	Initial (O) and Histology post-challenge (hours)	PC	BM/CT	PC	BM/CT	PC	BM/CT	BM/CT	BM/CT
1	5	(O) N/PVA	▲	N	N	N	▲	N	N	N
		18 PVA	N	▲	N	N	▲	N	▲	▲
2	7	(O) N/PVA	▲	▲	N	N	N	N	N	▲
		23 PVA/SVA	▲	▲	N	▲	▲	▲	▲	▲
3	8	(O) N	N	N	N	N	▲	N	N	▲
		12 N	N	N	N	N	N	N	N	▲
4	11	(O) N/PVA	N	N	N	N	N	N	N	▲
		22 N/PVA	N	N	N	N	N	▲	N	N

Key:
N – normal   PVA – Partial villous atrophy   SVA – subtotal villous atrophy
▲ – increased   BM/CT – basement membrane and/or connective tissue
PC – plasma cells

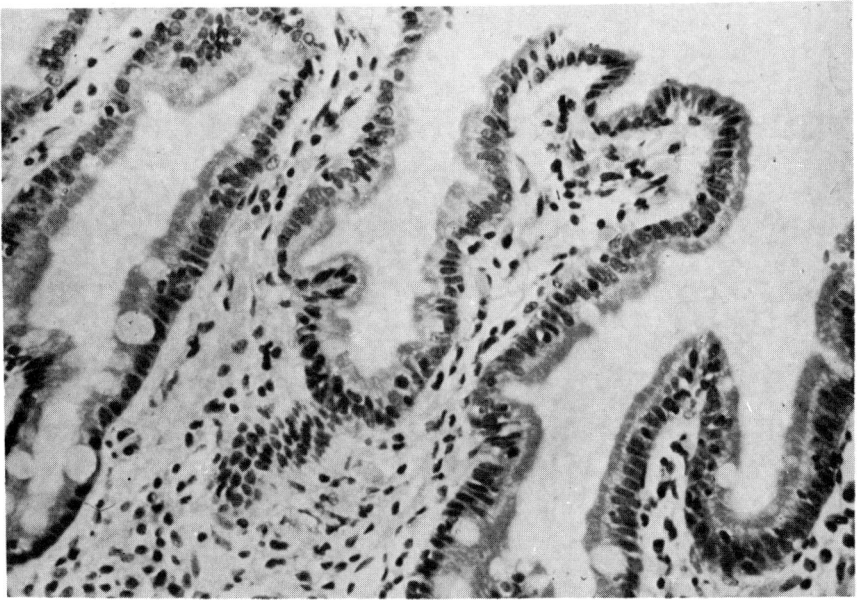

Figure 1. Villi from the jejunal mucosal biopsy of patient 2, three months after elimination of cow's milk. The biopsy was taken immediately before the milk challenge. H & E × 200

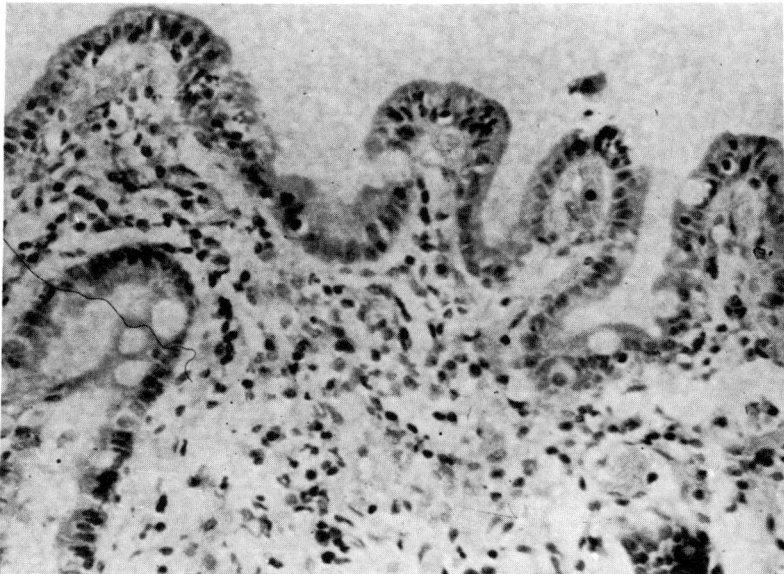

Figure 2. The mucosa of patient 2, 23 hours after cow's milk challenge. Compared to Figure 1 there is shortening and broadening of the villi, reduced villous epithelial cell height, elongation of crypts and intense inflammatory cell infiltration which includes interepithelial lymphocytes and polymorphs. H & E × 200.

TABLE II. Suspected cow's milk intolerance: electronmicroscopy before and after milk challenge

Ref No:	Age in Months	Biopsy: Initial (O) and after milk (hours)	Epithelium	Subepithelium	Inflammatory cells			
					Mast cells	Plasma cell activity	Eosinophils	Macrophage
1	5	0	N	N	N	N	N	N
		18	Lysosomes ▲ Vacuoles ▲ Mitochondria damaged	Oedema ▲ Endothelial Hypertrophy ▲	▲ *	▲	▲	▲
2	7	0	N	N	N	N	N	▲
		23	Micvovilli short Lysosomes ▲ Mitochondria damaged	BM Thickened Endothelial hypertrophy	▲ *	▲	▲	▲
3	8	0	N	N	N	N	N	N
		12	N	N	N	N	N	N
4	11	(O)	N	N	N	▼	N	▲
		22	N	N	N	▼	N	▲

BM – Basement membrane
▲ = increased
* Degranulated
N = normal
+ Polymorphs ▲▲
▼ = decreased

138

Electron microscopy (Table II)

Patient 1 – by comparison with the prechallenge ultrastructure there were changes in the post-challenge mucosa affecting the epithelium, the subepithelium and the inflammatory cells. The villous epithelial cells showed an increase in lysosomal and other smooth-walled vacuoles, and mitochondrial swelling with partial disruption of the cristae mitochondrales. The microvilli appeared unaffected. There was widening of the connective tissue spaces below the epithelium and this was presumably due to oedema. The endothelium of small blood vessels showed swelling and increased cytoplasmic vacuoles. Of the inflammatory cells there was an increase in degranulated mast cells, plasma cells showed dilated cysternae suggesting increased activity (immunoglobulin production) and an increase in eosinophils and macrophages. A few polymorphs were also noted.

Patient 2 – The mucosal ultrastructure, which was essentially normal before challenge except for some increase in macrophages, showed the most pronounced changes 23 hours after milk challenge. These were similar to those noted in the postchallenge mucosa of patient 3 but had additional cytopathological features such as shortening of the microvilli of the villous epithelium, thickening of the basement membranes of epithelial and endothelial cells and the appearance of dense translucent fibres, presumably collagen, in the connective tissue spaces. Numerous polymorphs and degranulated mast cells were seen.

Patient 3 – the ultrastructure of the jejunal mucosa was entirely normal both before and after challenge.

Patient 4 – the noteworthy features present in both pre- and post-challenge mucosa were 'inactive' plasma cells in which the cytoplasmic cysternae appeared in parallel fashion with opposed limiting membranes, and numerous macrophages with large phagocytic vacuoles which were partially filled with a dense homogeneous material.

Immunofluorescence of the jejunal mucosa (Table I)

In patient 1 an increase in IgG and IgE and complement could be demonstrated extracellularly after the challenge, and in patient 2, IgM and IgE were increased extracellularly, and IgE plasma cells were also increased in numbers.

Except for staining of basement membrane and connective tissue with antisera to IgA, patients 3 and 4 showed no overall change in the mucosal staining patterns when the pre-challenge mucosa was compared with their own post-challenge one.

Discussion

Our four patients had similar clinical presentations and did not react clinically to repeated small milk challenges – at least for the next 48 hours. Only two of these

139

(patients 1 and 2) showed morphological abnormalities after the milk challenge and these were similar when examined with both the light and electron microscope. Patients 1 and 2 also showed immunological changes within the jejunal mucosa after the challenge which suggested that though the types of immunoglobulins that were increased varied, IgE increases were common to both. These two infants also had evidence of serum complement activation 4 hours after the challenge.

Our preliminary conclusions are therefore that with the techniques employed we are able to detect which infants, in the absence of clinical reactions, are showing local (jejunal mucosal) reactions which can only be attributed to the milk. If this insult to the mucosa is allowed to go on it may well lead to chronic malabsorption and villous atrophy with obvious clinical manifestations.

The results in patients 3 and 4 show that over the period tested there was no evidence of immunopathological change within the jejunal mucosa. Does this imply that these infants are not intolerant to milk? The possibility exists that mucosal changes could occur after days or weeks. To test this, we reintroduced cow's milk to patient 3, who by our challenge tests was 'milk negative', followed her clinical progress over the next 3 months, and then repeated the jejunal biopsy. No clinical or morphological reaction occurred and we conclude that the patient was not milk intolerant. Patient 4 did not clinically improve over the next 4 months despite a milk elimination diet. Allergy to chicken meat was subsequently diagnosed.

Two recent textbooks of paediatric gastroenterology (Silverman et al, 1971; Anderson & Burke, 1975) have commented on the lack of rigid criteria for the diagnosis of milk allergy which would make this condition an acceptable clinical entity. In common with other investigators (Kuitunen et al, 1975; Walker-Smith, 1975; Freier, 1973) we doubt whether the criteria of Goldman et al. (Goldman et al, 1963) embrace all patients with this syndrome, since at least one of these, the return of symptoms within 48 hours after challenge, has been shown to be unessential. Anderson and Burke (1975) state that objective tests for milk allergy are as yet not available and that the diagnosis is in a similar state of uncertainty to that of coeliac disease before the era of jejunal biopsy. We should like to suggest that our method of detection of milk allergy, especially in the absence of clinical reactivity to a milk challenge, described in this paper, would provide this essential objective test. Of all the techniques described — histological, ultrastructural and immunological — we consider the routine light microscope preparation of the jejunal biopsies to be the most helpful for diagnosis.

In the differentiation of 'milk positive' from 'milk negative' patients our haematological data are unhelpful but it is possible that serum complement studies will prove of diagnostic significance. The increase in β-1a, a breakdown product of C3 complement, in patients 1 and 2 at four and five hours after milk challenge needs to be correlated with similar timed studies of the jejunal mucosa.

The relation in time between pre- and post-challenge jejunal biopsies is an important one. Most investigators (Kuitunen et al, 1973) have timed the post-challenge biopsy to correlate with the onset of symptoms which varies from a few hours to several weeks. We have chosen to re-biopsy within 24 hours of the challenge so as to minimise the effect of other factors, such as the introduction of different food antigens or intercurrent infections on the mucosa. We have demonstrated that within this short period when only cow's milk has been added to the elimination diet, severe pathological mucosal changes are seen. These occur as early as 11 hours but not at 6 hours after challenge (Shiner et al, 1975). It would appear that they continue for at least 48 hours after a single milk challenge (Walker-Smith, 1975).

Earlier work (Shiner et al, 1975) has shown that though the mucosa 6 hours after milk challenge showed only few morphological abnormalities (such as oedema and dilatation of plasma cell cysternae), there was evidence of increased immunological activity in the tissue, notably for IgM, IgA and IgE although not for complement. At 11 hours post-challenge, both pathological and immunological changes had occurred and these were similar in histology and ultrastructure to those mucosal changes noted in patients 1 and 2. Of particular significance was the heavy inflammatory infiltration of the mucosa, which included polymorphs, and the increase in mucosal C3 complement staining which was evident at 11 and 18 hours (patient 1) but not at 23 hours (patient 2). Increased mucosal IgE staining, and mast cell degranulation, which were thought in our earlier paper to be some evidence for local reaginic reactions, appeared common to all patients with the immunopathological mucosal changes following the milk challenge, but other immune processes were also demonstrated. The pathological basis of these suggested an Arthus reaction (oedema, endothelial reaction, thickening of basement membranes, appearance of collagen fibres and polymorph infiltration). These changes were not seen in patients 3 and 4 after milk challenge. We therefore suggest that milk allergy should only be diagnosed in the presence of jejunal mucosal immunopathological changes following a challenge with cow's milk.

References

1 Shiner, M, Ballard, J and Smith, M E (1975) *Lancet, i,* 136
2 *Paediatric clinical gastro-enterology* (Eds.) (1971) Silverman, A, Roy, C C and Cozzetto, F J, C V Mosby Co. U.S.A. page 182.
3 *Paediatric gastro-enterology* (Eds.) Anderson, C M and Burke V (1975) Blackwell Scientific Publications. Page 225.
4 Kuitunen, P, Visakorpi, J K, Savilahti, E and Pelkonen, P (1975) *Archives of Diseases in Childhood, 50,* 351.
5 Walker-Smith (1975) *Archives of Diseases in Childhood, 50,* 347
6 Freier, S. (1973) *Clinical Allergy, 3* (supplement), 597
7 Goldman, A S, Anderson, D W, Sellers, W A, Saperstein, S, Kniker, W T and Halpern, S R. (1963) *Paediatrics, 32,* 425
8 Kuitunen, P, Rapola, J. Savilahti, E and Visakorpi, J K (1973) *Acta Paediatrica Scandinavica, 62,* 585

141

Long-Term Management of Coeliac Disease in the Area of Berne, Switzerland

B HADORN, H GAZE AND U SCHAAD

Since 1968, 145 patients have been diagnosed as having coeliac disease. In all patients the diagnosis was confirmed by a small intestinal biopsy. Most of these patients adhered very well to the gluten free diet but in a few instances the diet was abandoned after various time intervals. In some of these patients clinical symptoms did not appear immediately and some had even lost contact with their physician or with our hospital. We decided therefore to review all patients regularly in our outpatient department. This decision was taken in agreement with the Bernese Association of Practising Paediatricians. During the same time interval approximately one hundred patients were referred to us by paediatricians not working in our hospital for reassessment. In this group of patients, the initial diagnosis had usually been made on clinical grounds only and no biopsies had been performed. The present study is certainly not the first of this kind but since it is a prospective study we feel that it is important to inform interested colleagues about the way the problem is dealt with in our hospital.

Management of patients

The management of the various situations is explained in Tables I and II.

Usefulness of the one-hour blood-xylose test

In 59 children who underwent diagnostic small-intestinal biopsies the correlation between the intraepithelial lymphocyte infiltration of the distal duodenal mucosa (Ferguson, 1974 and Figure 1) and the blood-xylose concentration one hour after ingestion of 5 g D-xylose was investigated. Sixteen patients with active coeliac disease had blood-xylose values below 20 mg %, and the correlation between blood-xylose levels and the numbers of intraepithelial lymphocytes in this same group of patients was found to be highly significant (see Figure 2). Provided that the methodology is meticulously followed, it is our experience that the one-hour blood-xylose test, in addition to the clinical investigation, facilitates the decision whether or not to perform a small-intestinal biopsy in the diagnosis and follow-

TABLE I

Group A no biopsy	at present gluten free diet or on normal diet for less than 1 year	gluten challenge
Group B no biopsy	on normal diet for more than 1 year	biopsy
Group C biopsy abnormal	gluten free	continuation of gluten free diet
Group D biopsy abnormal	patient has abandoned diet for more than 1 year	biopsy

means that decision about diet is taken according to the result of the biopsy

TABLE II Gluten-challenge

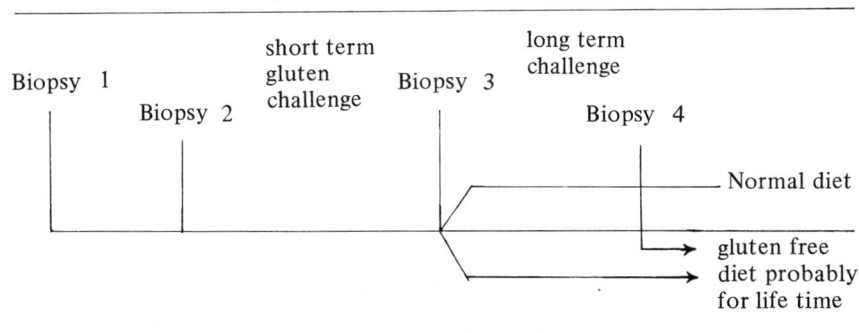

Biopsy 1   Biopsy 2   short term gluten challenge   Biopsy 3   long term challenge   Biopsy 4   Normal diet   gluten free diet probably for life time

1. In patients belonging to groups A and B (Table I) this biopsy was not performed. If biopsy 3 still showed a normal mucosa the child was put onto a normal diet. In this group of patients biopsy 4 was performed after 2 years unless clinical symptoms appeared earlier. The biopsy was also performed earlier if blood-xylose showed a tendency to drop.
2. 1 g/kg body weight per day boiled crude gluten* is added to a strictly gluten-free diet during 30 days.
3. Normal gluten containing diet.
* 'Aleuronat' purchased from Blattmann & Co., Wädenswil, Switzerland

143

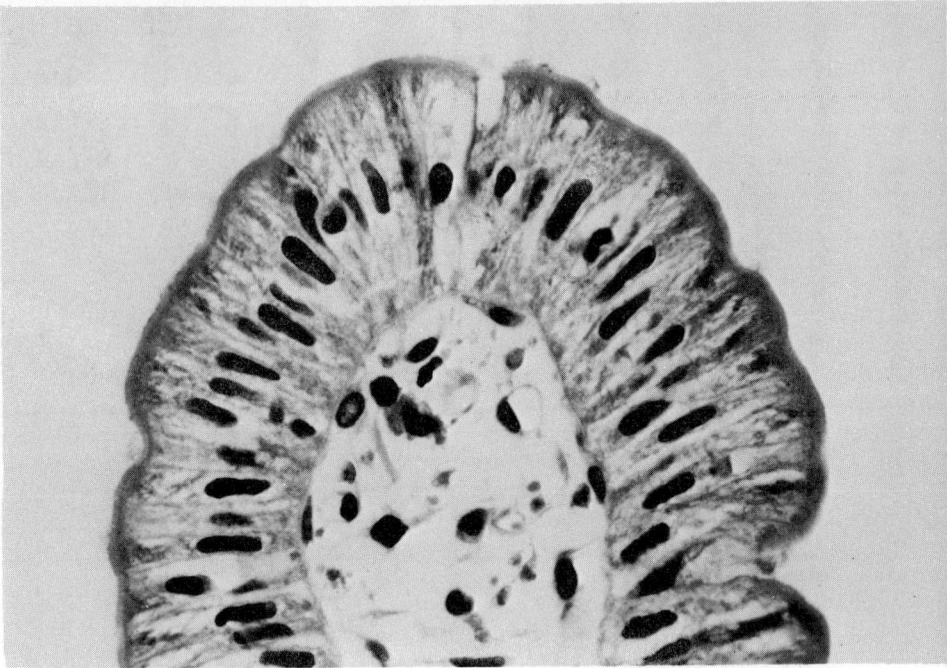

Figure 1a. Normal epithelium showing 3 intraepithelial lymphocytes

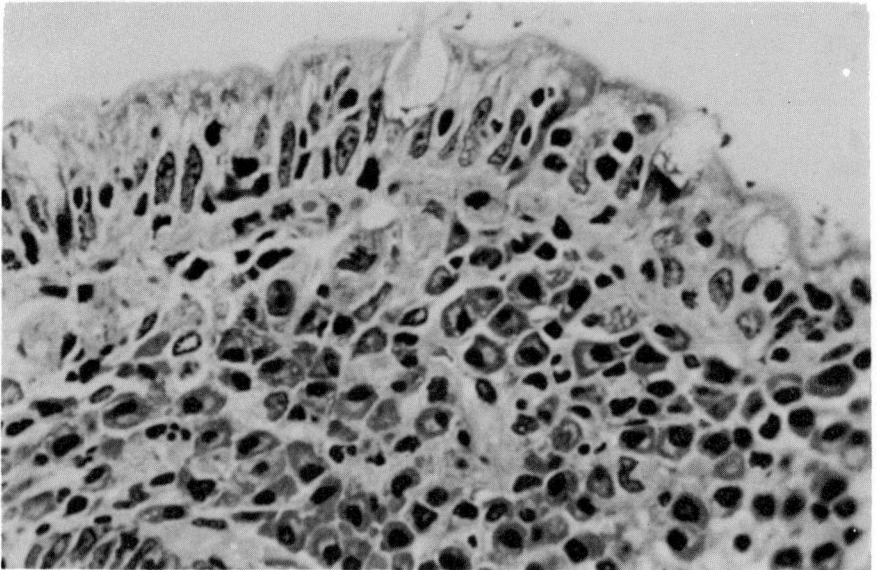

Figure 1b. Epithelium in acute CD showing 19 intraepithelial lymphocytes and plasma cells

144

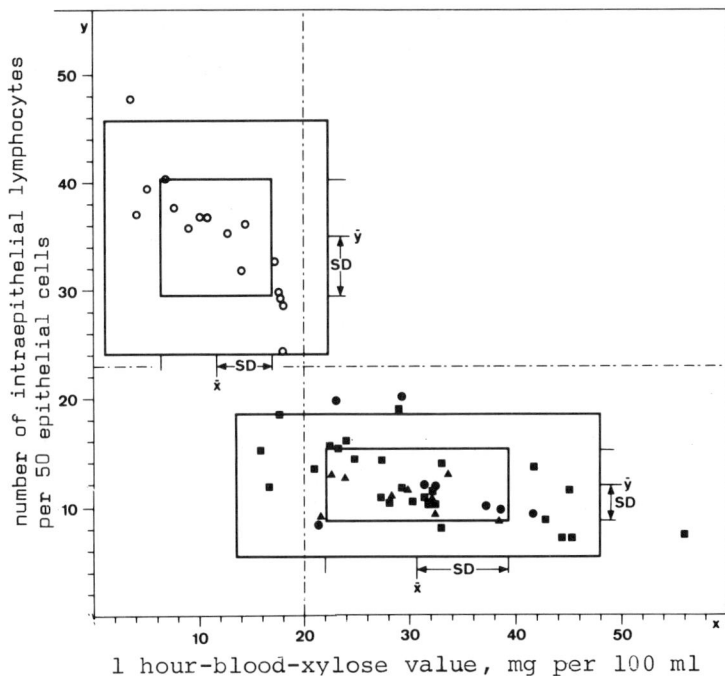

Figure 2. *Correlation between 1 hour blood-xylose value and number of intraepithelial lymphocytes* (from reference 2 with permission)

○ acute coeliac disease (CD)
● coeliac disease on a gluten free diet
■ clinical diagnosis of CD not confirmed
▲ control patients

SD = 1 standard deviation
(Schaad et al, 1975, with permission)

up of coeliac disease in childhood. The test however cannot replace the intestinal biopsy which remains the only acceptable criterion for the diagnosis of this disease.

Comment

During the short term gluten challenge the one-hour blood-xylose value was obtained in regular intervals. In patients who showed a decrease of this value a biopsy was performed immediately. In most patients exhibiting a decreased blood-xylose value an abnormal biopsy was found. This is in agreement with the observations made by Rolles et al (1975). A value of 20 mg per 100 ml was regarded as the lower limit of normal. However, if the blood-xylose showed a tendency to decrease, even values above 20 mg % were interpreted as indicating a slowly developing functional alteration of the mucosa.

145

Similar studies have been performed in other centres (Shmerling, 1971; Visakorpi, 1974) but we feel that a greater number of observations is necessary in order to decide if patients who have been diagnosed as having coeliac disease in early infancy will have to observe a gluten free diet during their life time.

References

Ferguson, A (1974) In *Coeliac Disease Proceedings of the Second International Coeliac Symposium.* H E Stenfert Kroese B V, Leiden (Ed) W Th J M Hekkens and A S Peña.

Rolles, C J, Anderson, Ch M and McNeish, A (1975) *Archives of Disease in Childhood, 50,* 259

Schaad, U, Gaze, H, Hadorn, B, Pedrinis, E, Cottier, H, Lorenz, E and Colombo J P (1975) *Helvetica paediatrica Acta* (In press)

Shmerling, D H (1971) In *Pädiatrische Fortbildungskurse für die Praxis, Vol. 30.* Karger, Basel. Page 86

Visakorpi, J K (1974) In *Coeliac Disease. Proceedings of the Second International Coeliac Symposium.* (Eds) W Th J M Hekkens and A S Peña. H E Stenfert Kroese B V, Leiden. Page 10

DR WALKER-SMITH Mary Harrison described a group of children we saw at Queen Elizabeth Hospital, London, who apparently had sugar intolerance following gastroenteritis. When they clinically recovered they were re-admitted and given a lactose tolerance test, which produced no diarrhoea. We went further and gave them 7 g of lactose per 100 ml, and feeding for 24 hours, and they still did not get diarrhoea. We then gave them a milk challenge starting with 5 ml of cow's milk and building up, and they then relapsed. In fact, some of these children then had excess reducing substances in their stools. We postulated that following an acute attack of gastroenteritis, in two cases enteropathic E-Coli enteritis, there was both lactose intolerance and cow's milk protein intolerance, but how they interrelated I do not know.

DR ROSSITER I wonder if I might add something to what Dr Walker-Smith has said? I have had two children with gastroenteritis and malabsorption, both about three months, one of them had a flat biopsy and the other a partial villous atrophy. The one with the flat biopsy had virtually no lactase, and the one with the partial atrophy, reduced lactase. Both these children were thriving on breast milk and on two consecutive days we gave them a test feed with milk. On the first day we gave them breast milk and lactose and on the second day we gave them cow's milk formula with the identical amount of lactose. After breast milk they had no symptoms at all. When they had the identical amount of lactose in the cow's milk, however, they had explosive diarrhoea with sugar in the stools. This presumably illustrates, although it does not explain it, the relationship between cow's milk allergy and lactose intolerance.

DR WILSON Dr Rossiter, do you think that if you were not giving lactose and you just gave lactose-free cow's milk protein, you would get as much in the way of clinical symptoms?

ROSSITER Well, very often of course the symptoms are not there. But I think more important would be to ask the question "Could lactose in the cow's milk challenge you are giving produce histological changes?". It ought not to produce the immunological changes which we know are there. I do not think anyone has really studied that possibility.

DR PROSSER When you have a coeliac child with a family history, do you think it necessary to do repeat biopsies on the child?

PROFESSOR HADORN I do not think that we can be sure, the genetics of coeliac disease are not clear. The inheritance of HL-A8 is important and this may predispose for coeliac disease as it does to other things. This may have an influence on the genetics of coeliac disease, and it looks as if it is dominant. I do not think that one can conclude that the form which the father has will be the same in the child. If the genetics were clear, then one could do that, but the genetics are not clear.

DODGE I wonder if anyone here has done HL-A typing in coeliacs and whether it might be itself an indication as to whether to do a repeat biopsy? It has been shown that 85% of patients with coeliac disease have HL-A8 and if you have a combination of apparent coeliac biopsy with a subtotal villous atrophy, and HL-A8, then the diagnosis is almost certain, so perhaps you need not go through challenging and so on.

DR McNEISH Always remember that 15% will *not* have HL-A8 and there is a recent report that there is no HL-A grouping that goes with cow's milk allergy, so that means that 30% with milk allergy are HL-A8, because that is the normal distribution. If you think a case might have coeliac disease then that case is that case and you do for that case what is required to exclude coeliac disease.

DR LEWIS Dr Shiner, in those patients in which you demonstrated marked C3 deposition in the mucosa, did you measure the serum complement and was there a fall?

DR SHINER We measured the β - 1a product which is a breakdown product of C3 and one would assume that if there is a change in C3 then the β - 1a should be going up. We found this in some patients but I must tell you that there are technical problems. Although we try in each case to take two or three different measurements, many times we get different results, and this problem has to be looked into. If I am talking about an Arthus reaction, it is much more on morphological grounds that we can be sure, than on immunological grounds, at least as far as C3 complement is concerned.
 Professor Hadorn, what is the average period between taking a biopsy and putting a child on gluten and then doing repeat studies? Is it variable?

HADORN Well, we saw some bridges and the villi began to show fusion and there was a great lymphocyte infiltration in the lamina propria and in the epithelium, but the villi were not flat.

SHINER Do you think it is enough to do just a blood xylose to evaluate

148

whether these children are coeliacs or not, or do you think you have got to do other things like taking a biopsy count of epithelial lymphocytes and so on?

HADORN We believe that it is necessary to do a second biopsy to show that they are on the way to recovery, but it may not be necessary to wait until it is complete.

SHINER And am I right in thinking that the patients you are challenging do not, on the whole, show a clinical deterioration over a period of two weeks?

HADORN Clinically, nothing at all, at this stage.

SHINER This is an important practical point, since it is said that one of the diagnostic criteria for coeliac disease is that when you challenge the child with gluten, it should relapse. This has been our experience as well, but many people still wait for a clinical relapse before they say it is coeliac disease and in the absence of a relapse, just will not recognise it.

HADORN I think that we and many others feel that in a very young child with coeliac disease, he will show clinical symptoms. In an older child, say from 4 to 5 years, there is much less clinical evidence of relapse.

SHINER Even more important than age, is the time which you have allowed on a gluten-free diet before you actually rechallenge. If this time span could be just 4 weeks say, then you will probably satisfy the criteria of a clinical relapse for coeliac disease, but if you allow several months to go on a gluten-free diet and then rechallenge, there is no clinical relapse.

DODGE I think this is possibly an area where there are differences between childhood coeliac disease and adult coeliac disease. My adult colleagues seem to feel that you are much more likely to get a prompt clinical relapse when you challenge patients with coeliac disease. I know we have one or two adult gastro-enterologists in the audience. Dr Mahoney, do you have any thoughts on this?

DR MAHONEY The challenge is usually accidental.

DODGE So if you make a diagnosis of coeliac disease, in adult patients, you normally do not challenge after that, but occasionally the patient inadvertently challenges himself?

MAHONEY Yes

DR HEATON I want to say I have no data on this, we do not normally rechallenge with gluten; as you say, they often rechallenge themselves. The trouble is they do not often in fact take a gluten-free diet. It is only recently that we have realised how difficult it is to get people to take a proper gluten-free diet.

McNEISH Martin Kendall, working in Birmingham with adult patients, has claimed that he can show a reduction in the urine xylose after gluten challenge in adults, very quickly, within a day or two, almost irrespective of the time they have been on a gluten-free diet. This is after they have been on an alleged gluten-free diet, but I agree with the other speakers that it seems likely that adults, in the main, are less well behaved than children and they are not usually on so strict a gluten-free diet. Whatever is the immunological component of coeliac disease, you might imagine that by regularly challenging it by small, frequent amounts of gluten, you keep that patient in an alert state, so that a formal challenge may give a rapid response. I think there is data in the literature to support biochemical evidence of speedy relapse of treated adult coeliacs, but how good their previous gluten-free diet was, I do not think anybody knows.

Abdominal Pain

Sources and Pathways of Abdominal Pain

JOHN S MORRIS

The majority of patients seeking the attention of a doctor do so on account of pain, and it has rightly been claimed that without pain there would be no clinical science and probably no doctors (Bockus, 1968). Despite the obvious clinical importance of abdominal pain, however, controversy still exists as to the mechanism of its production and of the neurological pathways involved in its perception.

In this brief review the various types of abdominal pain that occur will be described and the manner by which gastrointestinal diseases produce pain discussed.

SOURCES OF ABDOMINAL PAIN

It is now known that the abdominal viscera are pain sensitive although this fact was disputed until the beginning of the present century. The peritoneal coverings of the abdominal organs, together with the abdominal wall and the abdominal blood vessels are also pain sensitive. On rare occasions direct involvement of abdominal sympathetic nerves, such as occurs in carcinoma of the pancreas, gives rise to excruciating abdominal pain.

Pain is also referred to an abdominal site from disease in other organs and many children with pneumonia present with abdominal pain. Pain is also referred to the abdominal wall from lesions of the spinal nerve roots such as occur in herpes zoster and in tumours, primary or secondary, of the spinal cord.

Metabolic causes of abdominal pain must always be considered although in clinical practice they are rare. The best described metabolic cause of abdominal pain is diabetic coma or pre-coma but it must be emphasised that the diagnosis is a difficult one to substantiate and a laparotomy, if indicated, should be done once the keto-acidosis is controlled. Lead poisoning, porphyria and hyperlipoproteinaemia associated with pancreatitis are occasional metabolic causes of abdominal pain.

TYPES OF ABDOMINAL PAIN

Visceral Pain

An early denial that the viscera were pain sensitive came from observations by William Harvey on 'a young nobleman's heart' which became exposed following an injury to the ribs (Viets, 1957). Harvey showed that the exposed heart was insensitive to touch. Similar, but more extensive observations, on the insensitivity of the exposed human heart have been made in the present century (Alexander et al, 1929).

Observations with respect to gastrointestinal tract pain were not made until the advent of local anaesthesia which allowed the abdomen to be opened without interfering with any pain pathways which might derive from the abdominal viscera. Lenander (1907), in a series of observations showed that the intestine was insensitive to usual painful stimuli such as burning, cutting and pinching. By that time, however, it had been appreciated that pain could arise from the heart and it seemed likely that, in spite of Lenander's evidence, pain could arise from the intestine. Hurst (1911) argued that the stimuli that were used by Lenander were inappropriate and that there was no reason for the intestine to respond to stimuli to which it was not ordinarily exposed. As a result of a series of elegant experiments Hurst concluded that the only immediate cause of true visceral pain is tension within the muscle coats of hollow abdominal organs or distension of the peritoneal coverings of solid ones.

Despite the wide acceptance of the suggestion that distension of abdominal organs is the only cause of visceral pain there is some difficulty in explaining some forms of gastrointestinal pain. There is a very close relationship, for example, between the presence of gastric acid and the development of pain in patients with peptic ulcers (Dragstedt & Palmer, 1932; Bonney & Pickering, 1946). Hurst showed that the gastric mucosa was insensitive to acid so there is a seeming paradox in the observed relationship of peptic ulcer pain to gastric acid. Two theories attempt to explain this paradox. The first is based on the observation that acid induces reflex muscular spasm either around the ulcer itself or at the pylorus (Reynolds & McClure, 1922; Texter et al, 1959). The evidence in favour of this hypothesis is poor. The second and more acceptable theory is, however, that the presence of disease in the gastrointestinal tract lowers the pain threshold so that the mucosa becomes sensitive to stimuli to which it is ordinarily insensitive. Evidence in favour of this theory was provided by Kinsella (1948) who showed that the area around a gastric ulcer was sensitive to pinching and rubbing and by the observations of Wolf and Wolff (1947) on the subject Tom.

Neurological Pathways Involved in the Perception of Visceral Pain

The pain receptors of the gastrointestinal tract are thought to be unmyelinated nerve fibres derived from the autonomic nervous system found in the intestinal mucosa. These unmyelinated sympathetic fibres are known as C fibres and they transmit pain which is more diffuse and longer lasting than is the pain transmitted from the skin by A fibres. The conduction rate of pain impulses in C fibres is also slower than the corresponding rate in A fibres. The unmyelinated nerve fibres travel alongside the sympathetic nerves to the pre- and paravertebral ganglia and then enter the dorsal root ganglia at a synapse. The afferent fibres cross the grey matter of the spinal cord to a synapse for the second time. Afferent impulses then pass up the spinal cord in the lateral spino-thalamic tract to the thalamus where a third synapse occurs and the pathway ends in the post-central gyrus of the cerebral cortex (Figure 1). Within the lateral spinothalamic tract the visceral pain pathway is anatomically near to, and may be identical with, the pathway for somatic pain.

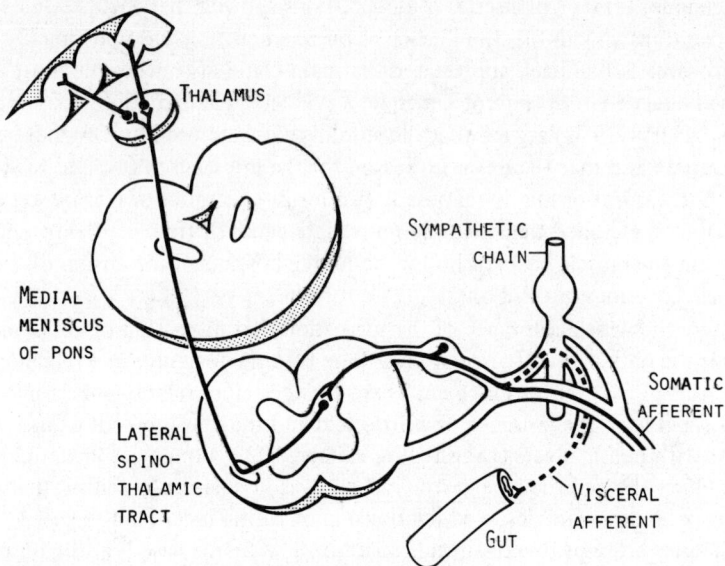

Figure 1. The neurological pathway of visceral pain.

The localisation of Visceral Pain

In a series of experiments in which balloons were inflated within the intestinal tract to the point of pain it was found that the pain was felt at or near the mid-line of the body (Jones, 1938) (Figure 2). The reasons for the poor localisation of visceral pain have been reviewed by White (1952). Since the accuracy of pain localisation is related to the number and overlapping of the sensory receptors it is clear that pain from the intestinal tract, which is poorly supplied with such receptors, is diffuse. In addition the ability to localise painful stimuli is dependent on the pre-

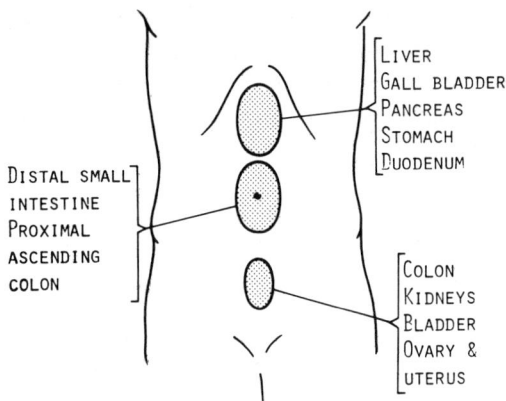

Figure 2. The localisation of visceral pain.

vious experience of the individual with consequent conditioning of the central nervous system. With respect to cutaneous sensation this localising ability is highly developed because of constant stimulation. Visceral pain, however, is experienced less frequently and the ability to localise it is not as good. Finally there is an anatomical explanation for the poor localisation of visceral pain, for the number of afferent visceral pain fibres in the dorsal root ganglion is greater than the number of fibres in the spino-thalamic tracts, so that impulses from different parts of the intestinal tract have to share a common neurological pathway.

Somatic Abdominal Pain

Disease processes within the abdominal organs ultimately progress to involve the peritoneal coverings and adjacent mesentery. The areolar tissue beneath the mesothelial layer of the peritoneum is richly endowed with nerve endings of cerebro-spinal nerves derived from the sixth thoracic to the first lumbar segment. Since these are somatic nerves the rate of conduction of pain impulses is faster and the ability to localise such pain is good. The result of any visceral disorder therefore, is first to produce visceral pain and then deep somatic pain. The classic example of such a sequence is acute appendicitis. In the early stages of the disease where obstruction to the appendix occurs the pain is central and around the umbilicus. As appendicular obstruction continues bacterial overgrowth occurs and inflammation develops in the appendix wall and peritoneal covering. The pain now becomes somatic and is localised in the right lower quadrant. The character of the pain changes and has a severe, knife-like quality—it is made worse by coughing and movement.

   Deep somatic pain is associated with other phenomena which include hyperaesthesia and muscle rigidity. The neurological pathways involved in the development of hyperaesthesia and muscle rigidity have been a matter of some discussion.

157

The earliest views were those of Mackenzie who doubted the existence of visceral pain (Mackenzie, 1909). Mackenzie suggested that noxious stimuli originated in the viscera and were relayed to the spinal cord where they set up an irritable focus which stimulated somatic sensory nerves. In this way all pain which derived from the gut, together with the associated phenomena of hyperaesthesia and muscle rigidity, were felt in the corresponding cutaneous site. If this were so these phenomena would have to be bilateral. Morley (1928) doubted that the autonomic nerves were involved at all in cutaneous hyperalgesia associated with deep somatic pain. He suggested that the nerves of the parietal peritoneum affect their cutaneous branches by radiation, the synapse between the two nerves probably occurring in the posterior root ganglion. Morley was less definite about the muscle rigidity that occurs in deep somatic pain but suggested that a true nervous reflex mechanism through the governing centre in the spinal cord is involved (Figure 3). Further work was done by Lewis and Kellgren (1934) which supported the work of Morley. They showed that these cutaneous phenomena were similar whether they arose from direct stimulation of the cerebrospinal nerves, the parietal peritoneum or the viscera. They suggested that the neurological mechanism by which these peritoneocutaneous and peritoneomuscular reflexes arise is by way of axon reflexes although the possibility that the spinal cord was involved was not denied.

Despite the large amount of experimental work and thought which has gone into the problem of these reflexes the neurological pathways involved remain uncertain.

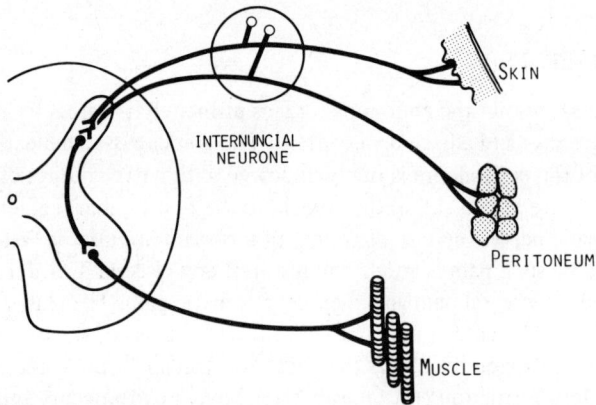

Figure 3. Reflexes involved in the development of hyperaesthesia and muscular rigidity.

Referred Pain from the Gastrointestinal Tract

In addition to visceral and somatic pain a third type of pain arises from disease of the abdominal organs. This third type of pain — referred pain — caused by reflex stimulation of the sensory branches of the phrenic nerve was described in a classic paper by Morley in 1925. Embryologically the diaphragm is formed in the neck and migrates caudally in early intra-uterine life. The diaphragm and the phrenic nerve are thus derived from the fourth spinal embryonic segment. In this way the central portion of the diaphragm and an area of skin over the clavicle the supra-clavicular fossa, the acromion and the supra-scapular fossa share a common inner-vation. Stimulation of this central portion of the diaphragm by perforation of a viscus, rupture of a solid organ or peritonitis thus results in shoulder tip pain. It is important to emphasise that this pain only occurs when the diaphragm is directly stimulated and does not occur in other upper abdominal disorders such as biliary colic. Shoulder tip pain does not seem to occur as often when the thoracic surface of the diaphragm is involved in inflammatory disease apparently because this part of the diaphragm depends less on the phrenic nerve for its sensory innervation (Morley, 1925).

Abdominal Pain in Common Gastrointestinal Disorders

The characteristics and causes of pain arising from disease of the gastrointestinal tract have recently been reviewed (Morris, 1973). Controversy persists over the true cause of pain in peptic ulcer but it is most likely caused by direct irritation by acid of an inflamed or ulcerated gastric or duodenal mucosa.

The development of upper gastrointestinal tract endoscopy has made gastro-enterologists more aware of the intense inflammation at the lower end of the oesophagus which accompanies the symptom complex of reflux oesophagitis. The reflux of gastric contents such as acid or bile causes pain in such patients (Bern-stein & Baker, 1958; Gillison et al, 1969). Reflux of gastric contents into the oesophagus does not depend entirely on the presence of a hiatus hernia and there is increasing evidence to suggest that the important factor is the competence of the lower oesophageal sphincter which is under hormonal control (Castell & Harris, 1970; Cohen & Harris, 1971). The association of cigarette smoking with dyspeptic symptoms has long been recognised (Gray, 1929; Edwards et al, 1959) and this may occur because smoking lowers the oesophageal sphincter pressure (Stanciu & Bennett, 1972).

Pain associated with the irritable bowel syndrome is probably the result of increased pressures within the small or large intestine. Such pain occurs frequently following a meal and it has been suggested that this occurs because the bowel of a patient with this condition is more sensitive to the hormone cholecystokinin which can be shown to increase intro-luminal pressure (Harvey & Read, 1973).

A large survey of randomly selected patients with and without gallstones showed that dyspeptic symptoms were slightly more common in those without stones (Price, 1963). It is unlikely, therefore, that gallstones, unless they pass through or are impacted in a bile duct give rise to pain. In some patients with gallstones there are disturbances of gastro-oesophageal and gastro-duodenal sphincter pressures which may explain the dyspeptic symptoms that occur in some patients (Capper et al, 1967; Johnson, 1972). It is unlikely that these pressure changes occur as a result of the physical presence of gallstones.

There is some dispute concerning the relationship between food intolerance and abdominal pain. There is a clear relationship between disaccharidase deficiencies in the brush border of the small intestine and the subsequent bacterial fermentation of sugars which cause gaseous intestinal distension and abdominal discomfort or pain. Dyspepsia related to fat however is not well substantiated. No relationship was shown between fat and abdominal pain in a survey conducted in an American hospital (Koch & Donaldson, 1964) or in a smaller controlled survey in the United Kingdom (Taggart & Billington, 1966). Physiological studies, however, have shown that the infusion of fat into the oesophagus lowers the oesophageal sphincter pressure, presumably allowing reflux to occur (Nebel & Castell, 1973). At the present time opinion with respect to fat induced dyspepsia is reserved. Patients with an irritable bowel syndrome often complain that their symptoms are more severe after eating foods such as tomatoes, cucumber or pork. A physiological explanation for these symptoms has not been found.

Abdominal Pain as an Expression of General Disease

The commonest general disorder which gives rise to abdominal pain is diabetic coma or pre-coma. It is often impossible to decide whether keto-acidosis has been precipitated by an acute abdomen or whether the pain is an expression of pre-coma, for there are no characteristic clinical features to the pain. The cause of the pain is uncertain; some patients have pancreatitis, possibly of vascular origin (Bossak & Joelson, 1956) and other patients in whom vomiting predominates have gastric distension. Hepatomegaly is a common accompaniment of diabetic keto-acidosis and it is possible that distension of the liver capsule is responsible for the pain in some patients.

The abdominal pain of lead poisoning is similar to that seen in acute intermittent porphyria. It is usually colicky in nature, vomiting is common and the pain usually centres around the umbilicus. Because of the neurological abnormality which accompanies each condition it is possible that the abdominal pain represents a disorder of intestinal motility although it is unusual for such patients to have gross radiological clinical or radiological evidence of intestinal obstruction.

Hypercalcaemia, of whatever cause, also produces abdominal pain. The pain is usually associated with acute pancreatitis and it has been suggested that calcium ions convert trypsinogen into trypsin (Haverback et al, 1960). Patients with hyperparathyroidism have an increased incidence of peptic ulceration which is a further cause of pain.

Hyperlipoproteinaemia (Types 1, 4 and 5) has been associated with acute abdominal pain due to pancreatitis. The cause of pancreatitis is uncertain although pancreatic xanthomas, impaired blood supply due to vascular sludging and fat embolisation from other sites have been suggested as aetiological factors (Greenberger et al, 1966).

160

Abdominal pain is also seen in conditions such as cardiac failure, uraemia and dissecting aneurysm of the aorta but seldom causes diagnostic difficulty in these situations.

Psychological Factors of Abdominal Pain

When all the usual causes of abdominal pain are excluded there remains a hard core of patients who elude precise diagnosis. Such patients are often thought to have psychological disease, although such a diagnosis is impossible to confirm and is a dangerous one to make. In an attempt to recognise psychological factors in patients with 'investigation negative' abdominal pain Hill and Blendis (1967) investigated a large series of patients. They pointed out the lack of objective evidence of organic disease and the high incidence of symptoms such as flatulence, nausea and vomiting. There was often a family history of abdominal pain and the patients often came from large families, and were, on objective assessment, neurotic. Many patients were depressed and pain disappeared when the depression was treated.

Psychological factors do not only induce abdominal pain but also modify the reaction of the patient who has abdominal pain of organic origin. Soldiers in battle with severe wounds often deny any pain at all, and sports injuries during the course of the game may also be painless. Such complex interactions between the psyche and pain perception only serve to make the proper clinical assessment of pain more difficult.

References

Alexander, J, MacLoed, A G and Barker, P S (1929) *Archives of Surgery, 19,* 1470
Bernstein, L M and Baker, L A (1958) *Gastroenterology, 34,* 760
Bockus, H L (1968) *Lahey Clinic Foundation Bulletin, 17,* 77
Bonney, G L W and Pickering G W (1946) *Clinical Science, 6,* 63
Bossak, E T and Joelson, R H (1956) *Archives of Internal Medicine, 97,* 201
Capper, W M, Butler T J, Kilby, J O and Gibson, M J (1967) *Lancet, i,* 413
Castell, D O and Harris L D (1970) *New England Journal of Medicine, 282,* 886
Cohen, S and Harris, L D (1971) *New England Journal of Medicine 284,* 1053
Dragstedt, L R and Palmer, W L (1932) *Proceedings of the Society of Experimental Biology (New York) 29,* 753
Edwards, F, McKeown, T and Whitfield A G W (1959) *Lancet, i,* 197
Gillison, E W, Capper, W M, Airth, G R, Gibson, M J and Bradford, I (1969) *Gut, 10,* 609
Gray, I, (1929) *Annals of Internal Medicine, 3,* 267
Greenberger, N J, Hatch, F T, Drummey, G D, and Isselbacher, K J (1966) *Medicine, 45,* 161
Harvey, R F and Read, A E (1973) *Lancet, i,* 1
Haverback, B J, Dyce, B, Bundy H and Edmondson, H A (1960) *American Journal of Medicine, 29,* 424
Hill, O W and Blendis, L (1967) *Gut, 8,* 221
Hurst, A F (1911) *Lancet, i,* 1051, 1119 and 1187
Johnson, A G (1972) *British Journal of Surgery, 59,* 449
Jones, C M (1938) *Digestive Tract Pain.* The Macmillan Company, New York
Kinsella, V J (1948) *The Mechanism of Abdominal Pain.* Australian Medical Publishing Company, Sydney

161

Koch, J P and Donaldson, R M (1964) *New England Journal of Medicine, 271,* 657

Lenander, K G (1907) *Journal of The American Medical Association, 49,* 836

Lewis, T and Kellgren, J H (1939) *Clinical Science, 1,* 47

Mackenzie, J (1909) *Symptoms and Their Interpretation.* Shaw, London

Morley, J (1925) *Clinical Journal, 54,* 617

Morley, J (1928) *British Medical Journal, 1,* 887

Morris, J S (1973) *British Journal of Hospital Medicine, 8,* 144

Nebel, O T and Castell, D O (1973) *Gut, 14,* 270

Price, W H (1963) *British Medical Journal, 2,* 138

Reynolds, L and McClure, C W (1922) *Archives of Internal Medicine, 29,* 1

Staniu, C and Bennett, J R (1972) *Gut, 13,* 318

Taggart, D and Billington, B P (1956) *Lancet, ii,* 464

Texter, E C, Vantrappen, G R, Lazar, H P, Puletti, E J and Barborka, C J (1959) *Annals of Internal Medicine, 51,* 1275

Viets, H R (1957) *New England Journal of Medicine, 256,* 702

White, J C (1952) *New England Journal of Medicine, 246,* 686

Wolf, S and Wolff, H G (1947) *Human Gastric Function.* Oxford University Press, New York

Peptic Ulcers in Children

J A DODGE

There is no difficulty in defining the essential characteristics of a peptic ulcer: it is a penetrating lesion produced in the mucosa and deeper structures of the alimentary tract by the digestive action of pepsin and hydrochloric acid. However, a number of distinct conditions are included in this broad category, with widely different aetiology, situation, pathology, clinical features and prognosis.

Aetiology

A superficial erosion in the gastric mucosa results from a breach of the normal protective mechanisms afforded by mucus and the rapid turnover of epithelial cells. In this circumstance, the apparent gastric acidity may be low because of back-diffusion of H^+ ions into the mucosa. Such lesions are an important cause of acute gastric haemorrhage in children, and usually heal very rapidly. A number of substances including aspirin, corticosteroids and cytotoxic drugs can produce this type of lesion, mainly by interfering with mucus synthesis. In strict terms, an erosion becomes an ulcer only when it penetrates to the submucosa, but aetiologically there is little or no difference between an acute erosion and an acute ulcer. The pathological appearance of a *chronic* ulcer is distinguished by the presence of fibrous tissue at its base. 'The development of chronic peptic ulcer is determined by the algebraic sum of two groups of forces acting upon the gastrointestinal mucosa, the one defensive and the other aggressive' (Sun, 1974). Some of the factors governing the secretion of acid, pepsin, and mucus are shown in Figure 1. In very broad terms, one might state that chronic gastric ulcer usually implies an impaired defensive barrier, whereas the aggressive effect of enhanced acid secretion is more often an important feature of chronic duodenal ulcer. Ulcers in the prepyloric region and the duodenum are epidemiologically and clinically similar.

In children, as in adults in this country, chronic gastric ulcers are much less common than those of the duodenum. There are probably no fundamental aetiological differences between childhood and adult ulcers, but the clinical features are considerably modified in children and are liable to be misinterpreted.

163

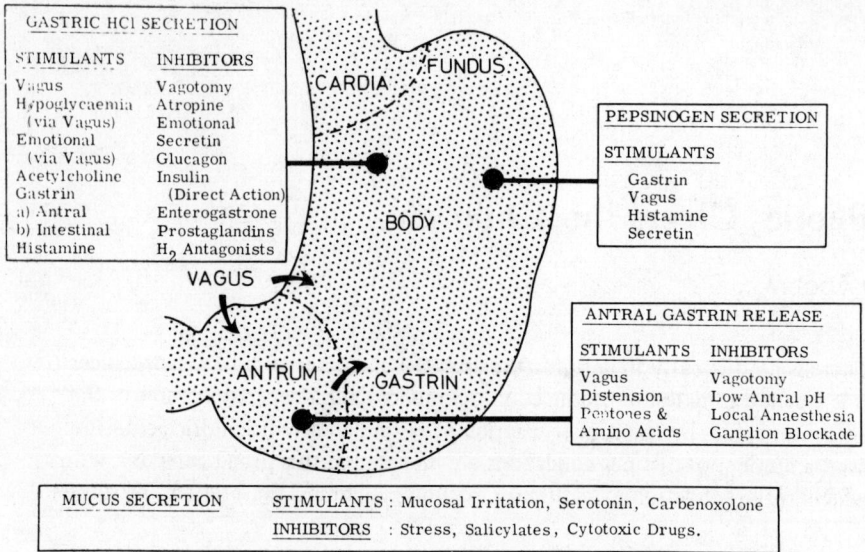

Figure 1. Secretory Function of the Stomach (Modified from Dodge, 1975)

There are several conditions which are associated with a relatively high incidence of peptic ulcers or acute mucosal lesions, but the site and chronicity vary to some extent. They may be responsible for initiating an acute lesion, perpetuating a chronic one, or exacerbating a recurrent ulcer (Table I).

TABLE I. Peptic Ulcers in Children: Clinical Associations

Aspirin
Burns
Corticosteroids
CNS Lesions
Cystic Fibrosis
Cytotoxic Drugs
Liver Disease
Pyloric Stenosis
'Stress': Infective, Traumatic, Emotional
Zollinger-Ellison Syndrome

I shall concentrate on some of the peculiar features of peptic ulcers in infants, and on the clinical picture of chronic duodenal ulcer in children, with a brief reference to ulcers occurring elsewhere in the alimentary tract.

164

PEPTIC ULCERS IN INFANTS

Shallow ulcers or acute gastric mucosal lesions are a not uncommon autopsy finding in newborn babies. They may be a terminal event in some cases, and are often but not always associated with a history of hypoxia. One estimate has put the incidence of such lesions as high as 25% (Watt, 1966), but this is not the experience of most authors. The true incidence of neonatal peptic ulcer is not known and is difficult to assess. Most instances described in live patients were brought to light by haemorrhage or perforation, and few of these infants had previous suggestive symptoms. In one series of 156 infants with peptic ulcers, 59 of them (38%) had perforated (Cosimano et al, 1960). In general, peptic ulcers in young infants are diagnosed in conditions of 'stress', including severe infective illnesses and after major surgery. The likely symptomatology of primary ulcers in the first weeks of life would be crying, vomiting, refusal of feeds and trouble-free intervals between these episodes: a syndrome familiar to all paediatricians, usually self-limiting and variously attributed to colic, 'spoiling', bad temper, maternal inadequacy, under-, over-, or improper feeding, and, in the older baby, teething. Nursing staff in Special Care Baby Units traditionally wash out the infant's stomach, presumably to get rid of the mucus which is thought to be responsible for the vomiting. But excessive mucus indicates gastritis, and may well be associated with gastric ulcers. Gastrointestinal bleeding, attributed to prothrombin deficiency and entitled 'haemorrhagic disease of the newborn', may also in reality be due to peptic ulcers or acute gastric erosions. There is certainly every reason why ulcers should be quite frequent in neonates. On the one hand, acid secretion is relatively high in the first week or two of life, presumably as a consequence of the surprisingly large number of parietal cells present at birth (Polacek & Ellison, 1966); while on the other side of the equation, the mucosal defences are probably to a considerable extent genetically determined and therefore vulnerable in predisposed individuals from the time of birth. The fact that most babies with appropriate symptoms soon recover makes full investigation unnecessary, and in any case radiological definition of ulcers is very difficult in young infants. Gastroscopy with suitably small instruments might be more rewarding, but is rarely justified except after a haemorrhage.

One association which has interested me has been between peptic ulcers and infantile hypertrophic pyloric stenosis. There are a number of case reports of the two conditions occurring together, and of course the uncommon adult hypertrophic pyloric stenosis is often associated with ulcers in or near the pylorus — the so-called 'pyloric channel syndrome'. It is suggested that in these adults, the ulcer produces pyloric spasm, and that this is followed by hypertrophy of the muscle (Burge et al, 1963). It is also interesting that an increased incidence of ulcers in later life has been described in patients surviving Ramstedt's pyloromyotomy in infancy (Steinicke & Roelsgaard, 1960). In my own series of 360 patients followed up between one and 18 years after Ramstedt's Operation, recurrent abdominal pain was present in 57. Only 17 of these were x-rayed, but of these 7 had duodenal ulcers and one had a lesser-curve gastric ulcer at the time of review (Dodge, 1974).

Mention should perhaps be made of neonatal gastric perforation. Although acute gastric ulcers perforate, many of the 'spontaneous' perforations seen in the first week of life appear to have resulted from ruptures of the stomach wall through congenital muscular defects. Predisposing factors include hypoxia, prematurity, gastric distension and trauma from nasogastric tubes (Shaw et al, 1965). Gastric muscular deficiencies are common in young infants, and the probable sequence of events is gastric ischaemia resulting from perinatal asphyxia, giving rise to localised mucosal necrosis and perforation (Touloukian, 1973).

DUODENAL ULCERS

Primary duodenal ulcers in children are probably more commonly missed than diagnosed. It is estimated that 5% of adults suffer from a 'peptic' ulcer, at some time in their lives, while of adults with ulcers, 2% give histories which date back from childhood (British Medical Journal, 1970). On this basis, a simple calculation suggests that the true incidence of chronic ulcers in children is 1 in 1000. The increased frequency with which childhood ulcers are diagnosed in recent years probably reflects greater awareness of the condition rather than a true increase. In adults, the trend is towards a decreasing incidence.

The case history of a recent patient with a duodenal ulcer will serve to illustrate a number of the important features of this disease.

> C.S. is 11 years old. At one year of age he was admitted to hospital after cutting his lip, and a diagnosis of haemophilia was made. His blood group was O.Rh.positive. At the age of five he was re-admitted with a history of abdominal pain of uncertain site, which was present for several months. A haematemesis and melaena had brought his haemoglobin down to 3.3 g. A similar episode a year later followed ingestion of aspirin, but a barium meal was normal. A family history of duodenal ulcer in his maternal grandfather and two other members of that sibship was obtained.
>
> Further gastrointestinal bleeding episodes necessitated hospital admission on three occasions, when he was nine, ten and eleven years old. On the last occasion a painless melaena stool was the presenting symptom. A repeat barium meal demonstrated a duodenal ulcer crater. Gastric analysis using pentagastin gave a Basal Acid Output of 3.5 mEq/ 10 kg/hr (normal < 1) and a Maximal Output of 11.2 mEq/10 kg/hr (normal < 3.5).

A highly selective vagotomy was performed 8 months ago, and he has since remained well. An insulin gastric analysis gave a BAO of 0.22 mEq/10 kg/hr and a MAO of 0.03 mEq/10 kg/hr when performed three months after the operation.

Genetics

A heritability of 0.93 has been derived for childhood duodenal ulcer, compared with 0.37 for adult cases (Cowan, 1973). Thus, a positive family history is frequently obtained. In one study of 46 children, 33% of fathers, 9% of mothers and 10% of grandparents also suffered from duodenal ulcers (Robb et al, 1972). Both these studies found the incidence of ulcers in parents to be about five times that of controls.

In adults, duodenal ulcers are more common in individuals of blood group O than would be expected by chance. A similar excess of group O has been observed in most childhood series, but, unlike adults, no excess of salivary non-secretors has been demonstrated (Habbick et al, 1968; Robb et al, 1972; Cowan, 1973). No significant difference between ulcer patients and controls was found when other blood group systems and eight marker enzymes were compared (Cowan, 1973). No completely satisfactory explanation has been given for the abnormal ABO blood group distribution.

The greater importance of genetic factors in the aetiology of duodenal ulcers when they occur in children may be accounted for in several ways. One suggestion is that environmental factors (such as smoking and 'stress') which are relevant in adults, have had less time to operate (Cowan, 1973). This is an alternative way of saying that the disease manifests itself at an early age simply because the child has inherited, in a polygenic manner, a particularly heavy genetic 'load'. His close relatives will obviously share much of his genetic predisposition, hence a number of them are likely to be ulcer victims themselves.

Clinical Features

A sex ratio of four males to one female emerged from the data on 791 cases collected by the Children's Peptic Ulcer Registry in March, 1974. There were seven times as many duodenal as gastric ulcers (R B Tudor, 1974, personal communication). In Robb's series from Belfast, the male preponderance was about 3:1.

The cardinal symptom is of course abdominal pain, but in children the pain is often atypical. It is mostly in the upper abdomen, but as often in the umbilical region as the epigastrium, and is the main symptom in over two-thirds of cases. The pain usually lasts for less than an hour, occurs once or twice a day, and comes in bouts with periods of remission lasting for a month or longer.

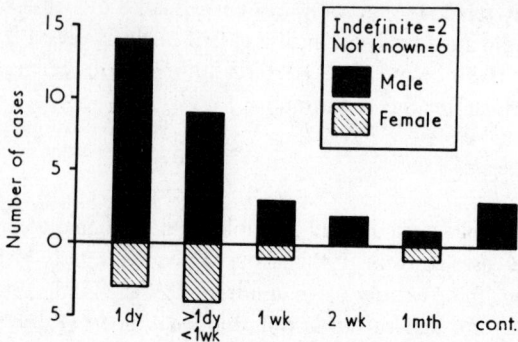

Figure 2. Usual duration of painful syndrome in 49 children with a duodenal
ulcer (From Robb et al, 1972)

The actual bouts are frequently as short as one day (Figures 2 & 3). The bouts
often persist for longer periods, and the remissions become shorter, before the
diagnosis is made, but by this time symptoms may have been present for several
years (Robb et al, 1972). A clear relationship between eating and pain is not
usually described, and night pain is present in a minority of children, although
when it does occur it strongly suggests the diagnosis.

<½ hour	½-2 hours	>2 hours	not known
19	19	3	8

Number of attacks of pain per day.

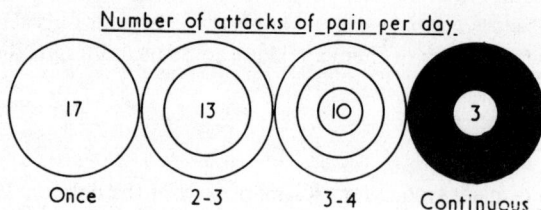

| Once | 2-3 | 3-4 | Continuous |

Figure 3. Pattern and frequency of pain in 49 children with a duodenal ulcer
(From Robb et al, 1972)

Vomiting occurs in more than half the patients, and is the presenting symptom in some. Nausea, water-brash and heartburn are other frequent secondary
symptoms and a few children complain of headache. The incidence of haematemesis and melaena varies widely from one series of patients to another, according to the method of ascertainment.

168

Several reviews have commented upon the high incidence of emotional problems in ulcer children, and this has also been my own experience. The importance of emotional tension as a primary aetiological agent is debatable; but even in young children acid secretion and mucosal blood flow are strongly influenced by emotional factors (Engel et al, 1954), and it seems inevitable that susceptible ulcer patients must be affected by these changes.

Investigations

Radiology

The demonstration of duodenal ulcers in children is even more difficult than in adults. Unequivocal features are the presence of a crater or persistent deformity of the duodenal cap, but filling of a crater may be very brief. Some radiologists and clinicians accept a number of indirect signs as probably indicating the presence of an ulcer: delayed gastric emptying, increased gastric secretion, pyloric spasm, irritability of the duodenum and coarse mucosal folds. The last three signs are often regarded as evidence of duodenitis, and may be found in adults (and children) with typical dyspepsia in the absence of a demonstrable crater. Presumably, it represents part of a spectrum of which frank duodenal ulceration is another part.

Children with such 'soft' radiological signs, or with no demonstrable abnormality, may show typical ulcer craters when a radio-opaque meal is repeated on a subsequent occasion. Where clinical suspicion exists, the diagnosis should not be abandoned until at least two negative barium meals have been performed.

Duodenoscopy

Modern fibre-optic instruments have brought the duodenum into the field of direct vision, even in children. In this country, success in diagnosing duodenal ulcers by this means has been relatively limited until now. This may be because of poor selection of patients for examination. In Cardiff, the incidence of peptic ulcer has increased considerably in the last twelve months (since our paediatric gastroscope arrived), but most patients were diagnosed radiologically. Increased awareness of the condition is almost certainly the real reason for the increase. The future will certainly bring further improvements in equipment designed for paediatric use, and, if experience in adults is any guide, endoscopy will be the most important diagnostic procedure.

Acid Secretion Studies

There is not much to be learned from acid secretion tests in children, unless achlorhydria or Zollinger-Ellison syndrome are suspected. On a weight basis, normal infants and children secrete about as much acid as adults (Table II).

169

TABLE II. Normal Values of Acid Secretion According to Age (mEq/10kg/hr)

	Basal Acid Output (BAO)	Maximal Acid Output (MAO)	Peak Acid Output (PAO)
Infants 1 yr	0.35−0.70	2.2−2.9	2.8 (mean)
Children 1−5 yr	0.35−0.95	2.4−2.6	4.1 (mean)
Children 5−14 yr	0.32−0.67	2.0−3.5	4.75 (mean)
Adults	0.20−1.00	2.0−3.5	2.0−4.2

(Data derived from various sources, particularly Baron, 1970; Dodge, 1975)

Children with duodenal ulcers generally seem to secrete more acid than healthy age-matched controls, but there is considerable overlap between the two groups (Habbick et al, 1968; Netakhata, 1970; Robb et al, 1972). Most reported studies in children have employed histamine or betazole as secretagogues, but the preparation of choice is now pentagastrin, 6μg/kg. Recent studies have confirmed that this dose, which is the same as for adults, is adequate to produce a maximal response (Becker et al, 1975). There is no reason to investigate gastric secretion routinely when a diagnosis of duodenal ulcer has been made.

Treatment

Current opinion is that neither dietary restriction nor antacids are of value in promoting ulcer healing. Nevertheless, symptoms may be relieved when the patient takes small, frequent meals, interspersed with doses of an antacid. Most children find a mixture of magnesium trisilicate and aluminium hydroxide acceptable, but it is worth ringing the changes with several antacid preparations if no relief is obtained or the child refuses to take it. A tablet containing milk solids and alkalis (Nulacin) is quite palatable and can be sucked unobtrusively in school. Naturally, the child should avoid specific foods which appear to exacerbate the pain. Adolescents should be advised not to smoke, because smoking decreases pancreatic bicarbonate secretion and delays ulcer healing.

Certain compounds are claimed to accelerate the healing of ulcers, but they tend to be more effective when the lesion is in the stomach. The most widely used is carbenoxolene sodium, which is said to decrease peptic activity, prolong the life span of gastric mucosal cells and increase mucus secretion. Side effects may be severe and resemble those of anticholinergic drugs. I have not ecountered these unwanted effects in children, but my experience is limited to a few patients who did not noticeably benefit from its use. Similar to carbenoxolene, but said to be less effective, is deglycyrrhizinised liquorice. A commercial preparation of this substance (Caved-S) also contains frangula bark and an antacid, and is well tolerated. Good results have also been reported from the use of colloidal bismuth (Salmon et al, 1974).

170

Other new approaches to treatment include an experimental trial of substituted prostaglandins (which inhibit acid secretion but often cause diarrhoea) and H_2 inhibitors, which block the receptors which are not affected by conventional antihistamines, and early experience of their use in adults has been very promising.

Surgery may be required for complications of duodenal ulcers, and for the intractable case where medical therapy has failed. Such children would probably come to surgery in early adult life, in any case, and there is no contra-indication to operation in childhood. Nothing is to be gained by postponing the decision to operate, and the patient may be spared years of misery. The operation of choice is highly selective vagotomy, without a drainage procedure.

ULCERS ELSEWHERE IN THE ALIMENTARY TRACT

Oesophageal Ulcers

Ulcers of the oesophagus occur in association with hiatus hernia, and this condition was considered in a previous paper (p. 83).

Meckel's Diverticulum

Meckel's diverticula are usually lined by gastric mucosa, and ulcers frequently occur either in the diverticulum or in adjacent areas of ileum. Bleeding is the usual mode of presentation, and it is often massive and painless. An important advance in diagnostic techniques has been the use of Technetium scans to demonstrate ectopic gastric mucosa (Kilpatrick & Aseron, 1972). After premedication with potassium perchlorate to block uptake by the thyroid, an intravenous dose of sodium pertechnetate ^{99m}Tc is given. After 30 minutes, abdominal scanning reveals radioactivity in the urinary tract, stomach, and, if present, other sites of gastric mucosa.

Jejunum

Unless the patient has had a gastrojejunostomy, ulcers of the jejunum are virtually diagnostic of Zollinger-Ellison syndrome. In this condition, a benign or malignant, non-β islet cell tumour of the pancreas produces gastrin, and massive gastric secretion of hydrochloric acid results. Severe, recurrent, intractable ulcers occur in the duodenum, stomach, and often the jejunum, with appropriate symptomatology. Diarrhoea is often present. Gastric analysis typically shows secretion of more than 100 ml in one hour, with a fixed acid concentration exceeding 100mEq/L and a high ratio of basal to maximal output (> 0.6).

In 15 children reviewed by Wilson (1971), six of the eight who had a total gastrectomy survived for more than five years, but six out of seven who had a lesser operation died of ulcer complications. All fifteen had gastrointestinal haemorrhage or perforation prior to surgery.

In children with recurrent ulcers, or a jejunal ulcer, it is worth bearing in mind that 5% of reported cases of Zollinger-Ellison syndrome have occurred in patients under 16 years of age.

References

Baron, J H (1970) *Scandinavian Journal of Gastroenterology, 5,* Suppl. 6, 9
Becker, M, Fritsch, W P, Hausamen, T U and Rotthauwe, H W (1975) *European Society for Paediatric Gastroenterology, 8th Annual Meeting, Brussels, April 11–12*
British Medical Journal (1970) *Leading Article, 2,* 583
Burge, H, Gill, A M and Lewis, R H (1963) *Lancet, i,* 73
Cosimano, S J, Jr, Lee J, and Balch, H H (1960) *Medical Annals of the District of Columbia, 29,* 13
Cowan, W K (1973) *Clinics in Gastroenterology, 2,* 539
Dodge, J A (1974) In *Modern Trends in Paediatrics, 4.* (Ed) J Apley. Butterworths, London. Page 237
Dodge, J A (1975) In *Paediatric Gastroenterology.* (Ed) C M Anderson and V Burke. Blackwell, Oxford. Page 653.
Engel, G L, Reichsman, F and Segal, H J (1954) *Psychosomatic Medicine, 18,* 374
Habbick, B F, Melrose, A G and Grant, J C (1968) *Archives of Disease in Childhood, 43,* 23
Kilpatrick, Z M and Aseron, C A, Jr (1972) *New England Journal of Medicine, 287,* 653
Netakhata, Z N (1970) *Pediatriya 1970/72,* 67, (Russian)
Polacek, M A and Ellison, E H (1966) *American Journal of Surgery, 111,* 777
Robb J D A, Thomas, P S, Orszulok, J and Odling-Smee, G W (1972) *Archives of Disease in Childhood, 47,* 688
Salmon, P R, Brown, P, Williams R and Read, A E (1974) *Gut, 15,* 189
Shaw, A, Blanc, W A, Santulli, T V and Kaiser, G (1965) *Surgery, 58,* 561
Steinicke, O and Roelsgaard, N (1960) *Acta Paediatrica Scandinavica, 49,* 4
Sun, D C H (1974) *Gastroenterology.* (Ed) H L Bockus. Saunders, Philadelphia. Page 580
Touloukian, R J (1973) *Clinical Pediatrics, 12,* 219
Watt, J (1966) *Journal of Pathology & Bacteriology, 91,* 105
Wilson, J H (1971) *Archives of Surgery, 103,* 108

Pancreatitis in Children

J R SIBERT

Pancreatitis was thought to be a very rare condition in childhood. Although not a common condition, it is not as rare as many paediatricians have thought. This is because many cases are looked after by general surgeons in peripheral hospitals, and many of these cases may go undiagnosed. Howat (1968) found 4 out of 54 cases of chronic pancreatitis had begun in childhood. Vernon, Stenning and Smith (1970) described four cases of chronic relapsing pancreatitis, which although diagnosed in adult life had long histories of abdominal pain going back to childhood. The prevalence of the condition in a British community appears to be one case per 500,000 children per year (Sibert, 1975a).

The majority of the literature on pancreatitis in children has been composed of single case reports; however, there have been four attempts to analyse its aetiological background. These have all looked at the problem in slightly different ways. Dobbs (1935) reported a case and reviewed the world literature of 14 other cases at that time. Frey and Redo (1963) report a large pathological post-mortem study from New York. Hendren, Greep and Patton (1968) reported cases from surgical experience in Boston and Moosa (1973) reviewed surgical experience over 11 years at Alder Hey Hospital in Liverpool. It seems from these and the single case reports that pancreatitis in childhood has many basic causes (Table I).

TABLE I. Causes of Pancreatitis in Childhood

Idiopathic
Virus infections (Mumps, ?Measles, Coxsackie, B,
    Congenital rubella syndrome, Influenza, Illness
    resembling Reye's syndrome)
Trauma
Hereditary
Drugs (Steroids, L–Asparaginase, Hydrochlorothiazide)
Pancreatic duct problems (Gallstones, Choledochal
    Cyst, Ascaris lumbricoides, ?Duct abnormalities)
Cystic fibrosis
Hyperlipoproteinaemia (Types I and V)
Hypercalcaemia
Malnutrition
Alcohol

TABLE II. Families with Hereditary Pancreatitis in the world literature

Name	Country	Aminoaciduria	Definite Case	Suspected case
Comfort & Steinberg (1952)	US	Yes	4	2
Gross & Comfort (1957) C Family	US	Yes	3	2
K Family	US	Yes	7	8
Gross (1958)	US	Yes	6	4
Cornet et al (1962) later added to by Bon (1971)	France	No	18	9
Gerber (1963)	US	No	2	6
Carey and Fitzgerald (1968)	Eire	Yes	3	8
Robechek (1968)	US	No	3	2
Whitten et al (1968)	US	No	1	1
Adham et al (1968)	US	No	5	2
Gross and Jones (1969)	US	No	2	3
Nash (1971) brought up to 1975	GB	No	4	2
Moretti and Nussle (1971)	Swiss	No	6	0
McElroy and Christiansen (1972)	US	No	10	16
Pestel et al (1972)	France	No	3	2
Kattwinkel et al (1973)	US	No		
West Virginia Kindred		No	9	21
Tennessee Kindred		No	12	12
Virginia Kindred		No	9	18
Edmondson and Holmes (1973)	US	No	7	1
Mott et al (1973)	Brazil	No	2	0
Bergstrom et al (1973)	Sweden	Yes	2	1
Scuro et al (1973)	Italy	No	4	1
Crane et al (1973)	US	No	3	1
Sato et al (1974)	Japan	No	3	1
Appel (1974)	US	No	3	4
Sibert (1975)	GB	No	9	15
McConnell (not reported)	GB	Yes	2	0

174

Many cases in childhood are *idiopathic*, and may be acute pancreatitis, relapsing pancreatitis or chronic pancreatitis. The majority of these children are in the older paediatric age group and may represent one end of the age spectrum of idiopathic, acute or chronic pancreatitis as it occurs in adults (Sibert, 1975a).

Mumps pancreatitis is a well recognised cause of pancreatitis in childhood, but it is a relatively rare complication of mumps (Eagles, 1947). *Other virus infections* have caused pancreatitis but more rarely than mumps. Coxsackie B virus infections have been implicated in infancy (Fechner et al, 1963). Pancreatitis may be a very rare complication of measles (Sibert, 1975b) and of the congenital rubella syndrome (Bunnell & Monif, 1972). Two papers from America have described the syndrome resembling Reye's Syndrome with acute encephalitis but with acute haemorrhagic pancreatitis rather than liver problems (Stover et al, 1968; Morens et al, 1974). In a paper from Poland, Swicowa and Mryglodowicz (1972) described 18 children with pancreatitis admitted to hospital in Gdansk (representing 13% of of all admissions for abdominal pain); 10 of these cases were associated with an influenza A2 virus infection.

Trauma appears to be a relatively common cause of pancreatitis in childhood, often with pseudocyst formation. This follows a blunt upper abdominal injury which may be relatively trivial. Bicycle handlebar injuries appear to be particularly liable to cause this problem on childhood. Child abuse may also cause this condition (Peña & Medovy, 1973).

Hereditary pancreatitis was first described by Comfort & Steinberg (1952), and now many families have been described in literature, particularly in the United States (Table II). It appears to be inherited as an autosomal dominant condition with incomplete penetrance. Patients get attacks of abdominal pain, starting in childhood and young adult life. The mean age of onset varies from family to family (4 years, Bon, 1971; 12.5 years, Sibert, 1975a). The attacks of pain vary from patient to patient and attack to attack. The severity of the condition varies considerably between families. In the family I described from the North East, only two out of 24 patients had really serious problems and none of the patients had steatorrhoea. In this family and in others in the literature from the case reports, the attacks of abdominal pain seemed to improve after the third decade. In contrast in the family which was described by Cornet et al (1962) and later by Bon (1971), all the patients seemed to have steatorrhoea and growth retardation, together with severe pain, sometimes starting as early as at 11 months of age. It is noteworthy also that the penetrance of the hereditary pancreatitis gene seems more complete in this French family. The families originally described from the Mayo Clinic appeared to have an associated lysine-cystine aminoaciduria. This has only been found rarely since and was thought by Kattwinkel et al to be probably a coincidental cystinuria in these families. Apart from the families described from the Mayo Clinic, only three other families in the world literature appeared to have aminoaciduria. The aetiology of hereditary pancreatitis is unknown. I know of five families in the United Kingdom with this condition. The families described in the world literature are shown in Table II.

175

Corticosteroid medication has been recognised as a cause of acute pancreatitis in children since Baar & Wolff described two cases in 1957. There have been several reports since them. More recently L-Asparaginase has been shown to cause acute pancreatitis, particularly in adolescent girls, during treatment of acute lymphoblastic leukaemia (Weetman and Baehner, 1974). Hypercalcaemia is a well recognised cause of pancreatitis in adults and has been described in children also. Jackson (1958) described a family with hereditary hyperparathyroidism and pancreatitis and Daum, Rosen & Boley (1973) described a 12-year old girl with acute pancreatitis and a parathyroid adenoma.

Conditions causing *obstruction or partial obstruction of the pancreatic duct* appear to cause pancreatitis in children. Gallstones, a very important cause of pancreatitis in adults, appears to cause some cases in children, but relatively rarely (only one case in the series from Hendren et al (1968) had gallstones, and none in Moosa's series). Children with choledochal cysts get recurrent pancreatitis on occasions (Gibson & Haller, 1959; Karjoo et al, 1973). Ascaris lumbricoides infestation has been reported to cause pancreatitis, probably by partial obstruction of the pancreatic duct. Three of Hendren's fifteen cases were thought to have congenital stenosis of the Ampulla of Vater. Shwachman and his colleagues (1975) have described 10 patients with cystic fibrosis who had recurrent attacks of abdominal pain diagnosed as pancreatitis. However, this does not appear to be a common complication of cystic fibrosis.

Families have been described wtih *acute pancreatitis secondary to hyper-lipaemia* (Kennedy & Collett, 1975; Poulsen, 1950). It is now clear that the types involved are Types I and V hyperlipoproteinaemia (Fredrickson & Levy, 1972). However it is noteworthy that patients with these conditions get recurrent abdominal pain without pancreatitis. *Malnutrition* appears to cause or to be an aetiological factor of pancreatis in childhood as it is in adults. Collins (1958) described from Africa four cases of kwashiorkor, which at post-mortem had pancreatitis. In several of Frey & Redo's cases at post-mortem in New York, malnutrition was also a factor.

I have collected cases of pancreatitis in children under the age of 16 years in the Newcastle Regional Hospital Board Area, retrospectively by ascertainment by the Hospital Activity Analysis (Sibert, 1975b); and recently collected further cases in a similar manner for Wales. I have now studied 22 children. Their aetiological background is shown in Table III.

One of the children died (a 13 year old with acute pancreatitis from County Durham). This is a mortality rate of 4% taking all cases and 12% taking just the acute cases. Both these rates compare favourably with the mortality rates of acute pancreatitis of 20% quoted by Trapnell (1972) and suggest that pancreatitis on the whole is milder in children than in adults. Pseudocyst formation was relatively common, 6 cases out of 22 (27%). Two of these had a traumatic aetiology and five were operated (the sixth case died). The three children with chronic relapsing pancreatitis form an interesting group. They all come from

176

TABLE III. *Aetiology of 22 cases of pancreatitis in childhood*

Idiopathic	11	
Acute	–	5 ⎫
Acute with possibility of 1–2 previous attacks	3	3 ⎬
Chronic relapsing	3	3 ⎭
Mumps	3	
Trauma	3	
Hereditary	2	
? Gallstones ? Idiopathic	1	
Measles	1	
Alcohol	1	

Wales; they have all had slightly suggestive, but by no means definite family histories of abdominal pain. Two of the children have had partial pancreatectomies and pancreatojejunostomies and have improved after this operation. The other child improved spontaneously at puberty. One of the patients had attacks of severe abdominal pain starting at the age of six years. He saw several doctors and was eventually referred to a psychiatrist in London. The diagnosis was not made until he was 14 years old and he improved considerably after surgery (Table IV).

TABLE IV. *Complications of 22 cases of pancreatitis in childhood*

Died	1
Malabsorption	1
Diabetes	2
Pseudocyst	6
Pleural effusion	1

Two children developed diabetes mellitus (one after a partial pancreatectomy) the other patient being the only one taking pancreatic supplements. There is no evidence of malabsorption in the other children, although they have not had pancreatic function tests. In fact all the patients are now thriving and in several obesity is a problem. It is noteworthy that two patients with acute pancreatitis were very obese adolescent girls, with normal serum lipoproteins. The one case caused by alcohol was a 14-year old boy who was given a litre bottle of cheap wine by a somewhat irresponsible father on a rare visit to the family home.

Investigations

The first step in making a diagnosis of pancreatitis in children is of course thinking of the possibility. The cornerstone in making the diagnosis is measuring the serum amylase during an attack of pain. Nevertheless, there are problems with this. Only 70% of patients with pancreatitis had a raised serum amylase on a single blood sample in one survey (Lifton et al, 1974) and therefore a normal serum amylase does not exclude the diagnosis. The serum lipase is traditionally thought to remain elevated longer than the serum amylase, but this has been shown to be incorrect (Trapnell, 1972; Lifton et al, 1974). However, the serum lipase is of value in raising the detection rate of pancreatitis from 70 to 83% if taken in conjunction with the serum amylase. It is also of value in detecting mumps pancreatitis, as the serum amylase is raised from the salivary enzyme in this condition. The urinary amylase may remain elevated longer than the serum enzyme and is therefore of value if the diagnosis is in doubt. Hyperamylasaemia is found in ketoacidosis, in renal failure and in macroamylasaemia. Therefore care should be taken in interpreting a raised value. Macroamylasaemia is an ill-understood condition of probably varied aetiology and is due to complexing of the serum amylase to a high molecular weight protein. This gives a low amylase clearance and normal urinary values with raised serum amylase levels (Berk, Fridhandler & Montgomery, 1973). Naturally enough the serum amylase is usually estimated in patients with abdominal pain, and therefore most patients described with macroamylasaemia have such pain. However, patients have been described without abdominal pain (Imrie, King & Henderson, 1973). Recently, we have had a boy with recurrent upper abdominal pain, which is probably of psychological origin. He had persistently raised serum amylase level with normal urinary values. This amylase is probably linked to his IgG and, interestingly enough, he has recently developed a goitre due to Hashimoto's thyroiditis.

The traditional teaching that laparotomy is harmful in pancreatitis has been challenged (Trapnell & Anderson, 1967). The authors found almost identical mortality in those cases which had conservative treatment, and those who had immediate laparotomy (20% and 21%). In childhood where there is always more doubt about the diagnosis than with adults, because of its relative rarity; it may therefore be worth considering laparotomy as a diagnostic measure. However, it is noteworthy that outside the acute attack, the pancreas may feel normal at laparotomy in relapsing acute pancreatitis, such as hereditary pancreatitis. In a similar way, although pancreatic function tests, such as Lundh meal, will be abnormal in chronic pancreatitis, it is worth remembering that again they may be normal in relapsing acute pancreatitis between attacks.

Treatment

Treatment of the acute attack is basically pain relief and fluid replacement. Apart from diagnostic reasons, there seems little place for elective surgery at this time (Trapnell, 1972). The role of the trypsin inhibiter aprotinin (Trasylol) is contro-versial. Nardi (1963) found no benefit from its use. However, Trapnell et al (1974) found some evidence that it reduced mortality in acute pancreatitis. Two patients in my series and many patients with hereditary pancreatitis in the litera-ture had some successful results from pancreatojejunostomies. Nevertheless, it is worth remembering that other children with chronic pancreatitis and many patients with hereditary pancreatitis, undergo spontaneous remission in their teenage years, and most attacks of pancreatitis resolve spontaneously without the need of any treatment, and often may be relatively mild.

Conclusion

Pancreatitis in childhood is a rare condition of varied aetiology. Although rare, it is relatively easy to screen for during an acute attack, and its early detection can be very valuable to the patient.

References

Asham, N F, Dyce, B and Haverback, B J (1968) *American Journal of Digestive Diseases, 13,* 8

Appel, M F (1974) *Archives of Surgery, 108,* 63

Baar, H S and Wolff, O H (1957) *Lancet, i,* 812

Bergström, K, Hellstrøm, K, Kallner, M and Lundh, G (1973) *Scandinavian Journal of Gastroenterology, 8,* 217

Berk, J L, Fridhandler, L and Montgomery, K (1973) *Gut, 14,* 726

Bon, G (1971) *Les Pancréatites chroniques familiales. Thèse pour le Doctorat en Médecine.* Université de Nantes.

Bunnell, C E and Monif, G R G (1972) *Journal of Pediatrics, 80,* 465

Carey, M C and Fitzgerald, O (1968) *Gut, 9,* 700

Collins, J (1958) *Archives of Disease in Childhood, 33,* 432

Comfort, M W and Steinberg, A G (1952) *Gastroenterology, 21,* 54

Cornet, E, Dupon, H, Hardy, M and Gordeef, A (1962) *Journal de chirurgie, 84,* 527

Crane, J M, Amoury, R A and Hellerstein, S C (1973) *Journal of Pediatric Surgery, 8,* 893

Daum, F, Rosen, J F and Boley, S C (1973) *Journal of Pediatrics, 83,* 275

Davidson, P, Contanza, D, Swieconek, J A and Harris, J B (1968) *Annals of Internal Medicine, 68,* 88

Dobbs, R H (1935) *Lancet, ii,* 989

Eagles, A Y (1947) *Archives of Internal Medicine, 80,* 374

Edmondson, H T and Holmes, W C (1973) *Journal of the Medical Association of Georgia, 62,* 137

Fechner, R E, Smith, M G and Middlekamp, J N (1963) *American Journal of Pathology, 42,* 493

Fredrickson, D S and Levy, R I (1972) *Metabolic Basis of Inherited Disease. 3rd Edn.* (Ed) J B Stanbury, J B Wyngaarden and D S Fredrickson. McGraw-Hill, New York

Frey, C and Redo, S F (1963) *Pediatrics, 32,* 93

Gerber, B C (1963) *Archives of Surgery, 87,* 70

Gibson, L E and Haller, J A (1959) *Journal of Pediatrics, 55,* 650

Gross, J B (1958) *Annals of Internal Medicine, 49,* 796

Gross, J B, Gambill, E E and Ulrich, J A (1962) *American Journal of Medicine, 33,* 358

Gross, J B, Ulrich, J A and Maher, F T (1961) *Further Observations on the Hereditary Form of Pancreatitis. The Exocrine Pancreas.* CIBA Foundation Symposium. (Ed) A V S de Reuck and M P Cameron. Little, Brown & Co, Boston. Page 278

Gross, J B and Jones, J D (1971) *Hereditary Pancreatitis. Analysis of Experience to May 1969. The Exocrine Pancreas.* (Ed) I T Beck and D G Saunders. J A Churchill, London. Page 247

Hendren, W H, Greep, J M and Patton, A S (1968) *Archives of Disease in Childhood, 40,* 132

Howat, H T (1968) *Postgraduate Medical Journal, 44,* 733

Imrie, C W, King, J and Henderson, A R (1973) *Scottish Medical Journal, 18,* 188
Jackson, C E (1958) *Annals of Internal Medicine, 49,* 879
Karjoo, M, Bishop, H C, Borns, P and Holtzapple, P G (1973) *Pediatrics, 51,* 289
Kattwinkel, J, Lapey, J, di Sant'Agnese, P A and Edwards, W A (1973) *Pediatrics, 51,* 55
Kennedy, R C J and Collett, R W (1947) *American Journal of Diseases of Children, 78,* 80
Lifton, L J, Slickers, K A, Pragay, D A and Katz, L A (1974) *Journal of the American Medical Association, 229,* 47
Logan, A, Schlicke, C P and Manning, G B (1968) *American Journal of Surgery, 115,* 112
McElroy, R and Christiansen, R A (1972) *American Journal of Medicine, 52,* 228
Moosa, A R (1973) *Progress in Paediatric Surgery, 4.* University Park Press, Baltimore.
Morens, D M, Hammar, S L and Heicher, D A (1974) *American Journal of Diseases of Children, 128,* 40
Moretti, G E and Nussle, D (1971) *Schweizerische medizinische Wochenschrift, 101,* 602
Mott, C de B, Bove, P, Ohki, Y, Conte, V P, Machado, M C C and Bettarello, A (1973) *Arquiva Gastroenterologia, São Paulo, 10,* 211
Nardi, G C (1963) *Lancet, ii,* 1065
Nash, F W (1971) *Proceedings of the Royal Society of Medicine, 64,* 17
Peña, S D J and Medovy, H (1973) *Journal of Pediatrics, 83,* 1026
Pestel, M, Lambert, C, Estenne, B and Estenne, M (1972) *Annales de médecine Interne, 123* 481
Poulsen, H M (1950) *Acta Medica Scandinavica, 138,* 413
Robacher, P J (1969) *American Journal of Surgery, 113,* 819
Sato, T and Saitoh, Y (1974) *American Journal of Surgery, 127,* 511

Recurrent Abdominal Pain

A Physician's Views

J APLEY

How common is recurrent abdominal pain, all over the world? My 'Index of National Sophistication' indicates that *'The more sophisticated the country, the more bellyachers will it have, large or small'.*

Do children with recurrent abdominal pain 'grow out of it'? We carried out a survey in Bristol some years ago and the answer was that, untreated, many did not. Does treatment help them to do so? In other words, 'Do little bellyachers grow up to be big bellyachers' in spite of anything doctors can do? Recurrent abdominal pain is one of the commonest childhood complaints, affecting 1 in 9 unselected schoolchildren in England (Apley & Naish, 1958). An organic cause is found in only a small proportion of them, hardly more than 1 in 20 (Apley, 1975). It is with a group of the *non*-organic cases, the 19 out of 20, that this paper is mainly concerned. The interesting but individually rare organic causes are discussed in my monograph.

To remind us of what sort of children have recurrent abdominal pain here is a summary, based on many hundreds of cases over many years (Table I).

TABLE I. Recurrent Abdominal Pain : Clinical Profile

THE WHOLE CHILD
    History: recurrent disorders
    Physique: slightly underweight
    Intelligence: normal
    Psyche: emotional disturbances
    Personality: timid, anxious, over-conscientious

THE WHOLE FAMILY
    Recurrent pains (head, abdomen, etc.)
    Nervous disorders

I had previously followed up a series of 30 patients with recurrent abdominal pain given a bottle of medicine or virtually untreated, and this will be used as a basis for comparison. The new series I am now reporting was also studied in

Bristol, nearly all by interviews in the homes (with the parents taking part in 15 cases) by one of my colleagues, to assess whether the sort of treatment we attempted, as children's doctors, can alter the prognosis in the long term.

All our treatment consisted of was reassurance, based on a knowledge of child and family, and on simple explanations and discussions; no drugs were used, and I know no other useful treatment. You can look up the details in *The Child with Abdominal Pains* (Apley, 1975).

THE TWO SERIES COMPARED

Each series consisted of 30 patients. All the children had been referred for recurrent abdominal pain to a paediatrician at Bristol Children's Hospital. There were three criteria for inclusions in either study: at least three episodes of pain, over a period longer than three months, severe enough to affect the child's activities. The original numbers collated in both series were about twice as large, but a considerable number, especially of older patients, had left the parental home when they grew up and could not be traced. (A few had come from abroad and a few more did not comply exactly with the criteria. A further three cases were excluded from each series because the patients seemed seriously disturbed and it was considered advisable to refer them on for psychiatric treatment.)

The groups were made up almost equally of boys and girls. The length of the follow-up period was from 8 to 20 years in the untreated series and from 10 to 14 years in the treated group. The ages of the patients at the time of the follow-up were 15 and 24 years in the first and 15 to 28 years in the second series.

Four Questions to be Answered

1) What happens regarding the abdominal pains as such? Do children grow out of them?
2) Are the patients liable to other disorders later in life?
3) Do the patients live ordinary lives when they grow up?
4) What factors influence the prognosis?

Do Children 'Grow out of them'?

In 19 of 30 treated cases abdominal pains ceased; 14 quickly after treatment started and 5 later. In the remaining 11, pains of some degree continued into adolescent or early adult life, which was as far as the survey could be taken. These bald figures are far from showing the whole picture; but so far as this statement goes they are almost identical with those of the earlier, untreated series (Table II).

So, in both series just under one third of the children became symptom-free. Let us now compare those remaining, those who grew up with abdominal or/and other symptoms.

182

TABLE II. *Untreated v. Treated*

At follow-up	Previous 'untreated' series	Present 'treated' series
No abdominal pains, no other symptoms	9	9
No abdominal pains, but other symptoms	9	10
Abdominal pains continuing with other systems	12	11

What Happens with the Abdominal Pains?

If there is no change in *quantity,* what about *quality* of the pains? In 11 of the treated series attacks of abdominal pain persisted into adolescence or early adult life. In 7 they were mild and infrequent. In 2 moderate and less frequent and in 2 they continued to be severe and frequent (Table III).

On the whole, in cases where the pains disappeared they did so more quickly in the treated series.

TABLE III. *Follow-up of 30 Treated Cases*

Description of pains	Number
No pains (rapidly ceased 13) (slowly ceased 6)	19
mild and infrequent	7
moderate, less frequent	2
severe and frequent	2*

*In one of the 2 severe cases with continuing pain the patient lost weight and in early adult life a depressive state was diagnosed. In the other, at 21 years bilateral ovarian cysts were found, and I shall refer again to this.

Is the Patient Liable to Other Disorders Later in Life?

We can compare the untreated and the treated groups (Table IV).

TABLE IV. *Follow-up : Other Disorders*

		Untreated	Treated
Pains	Migraine	3	0
	Headaches	15	3
	Other pains	4	5
	Other disorders	5	6
Nervous disorders		13	6
Organic disease		1	1

It can be seen that, as regards other disturbances, the treated cases did much better than the untreated.

Do the Patients Live Ordinary Lives when They Grow up?

We can now see how the patients lived with their troubles (Table V).

TABLE V. Follow-up of 21 Treated Cases

Abdominal pains	Work and other activities	
	restricted	not restricted
none	–	10
mild or moderate	–	9
severe and frequent	2	–

In all but the two severe cases, the patients learned to understand and accept the association of stress and pain. In all but these two, their symptoms did not cause absenteeism from work or interfere with their activities. I cannot compare these results exactly with the untreated series. People do sometimes learn from experience, and *we* learned to ask more profound questions. But in the untreated series we estimated that nearly half the cases followed were not well adapted and did *not* live reasonably normal lives.

What Factors Influence the Prognosis?

1. In children from 'Painful Families' (i.e. one or both parents with recurrent pains, together with seriously disturbed families), the pains are more likely than in more normal families to persist and to be associated with anxiety.

2. Girls have a better chance than have boys that the abdominal pains will cease, but a rather higher chance of developing other symptoms.

3. If pains start after six years of age, there is a slightly greater chance of complete recovery and a slightly lower incidence of extra-abdominal symptoms.

4. The prognosis is much better in patients whose symptoms had occurred for less than six months before we treated them. This is like leukaemia in childhood. The longer it goes on, without proper treatment, the harder it is to treat effectively (Table VI).

A boy, under six, of a 'painful family', not treated fairly promptly, would have a bleak prognosis.

184

TABLE VI. Good and Bad Prognostic Points

Factor	Prognosis better	Prognosis worse
family	normal	'painful family'
sex	female	male
age of onset	over 6 years	under 6 years
period before treatment	under 6 months	over 6 months

Discussion

I shall say something about a few interesting points: organic disease, acute appendicitis, psychiatric disease, 'painful families' and research on the reactions of the pupils in little bellyachers.

Organic Disease

When psychosomatic disorders are diagnosed the doctor may secretly fear that, despite all precautions, he is overlooking organic disease. The two series discussed here together comprise 60 cases who were followed up for many years. Among these 60, one undiagnosed organic disorder did come to light subsequently. This was in a female with mainly right-sided pain who proved to have dermoid cysts of both ovaries. She had been investigated more exhaustively than any other patient, partly because of my guiding rule worked out from our experience that: *'The further the pains are from the centre, the more likely they are to be due to organic disease'.* One *untreated* case later had a duodenal ulcer.

With rare exceptions organic disease can be ruled out from a carefully taken history, when it is a history appropriate to the disorder, together with a minimum of investigations (only one test is *always* mandatory: a thorough urine examination). Two facets of diagnosis are necessary and complementary: reasonable evidence against organic disease, together with evidence in favour of an emotional disturbance. It is wise not to rely on one alone, but to have both. If improvement does not occur, either the emotional or physical aspects can, of course, be examined further — but over-investigation has its own dangers.

Appendicitis

The clinical diagnosis of acute appendicitis in children is notoriously fraught with difficulty, and where genuine doubt exists it is clearly safer to operate. Moreover, if the pains continue afterwards, the doctor is comforted by knowing that he is not overlooking a potentially dangerous condition. It seems, however, most unlikely that recurrent or chronic appendicitis can cause frequent attacks of pain

185

over a period of many months or years. My practice is to advise against operation unless, during an attack, there is anorexia, pain on movement and preferably evidence of localisation of pain, together with definite tenderness and resistance, in the right iliac fossa. I consider the crucial feature in diagnosis to be a change in symptomatology.

Psychiatric Disease

There have been claims that recurrent abdominal pain in childhood is commonly a manifestation of depressive illness, and so recurrent abdominal pain may be treated with anti-depressive drugs. In our experience depression, at the time or later in life, is not common. At the most, one in ten cases may be so labelled. A far commoner factor is anxiety.

Painful Families

The present series has confirmed the high incidence of 'painful families', families with frequent pains as previously described. The family pains were mainly abdominal: in 11 of 30 cases one (or occasionally both) parents had abdominal symptoms. Pains elsewhere, and migraine, were common too, and 'nerves' even commoner. We have learned to ask twice — and find many more parents have migraine on the second asking.

The child with recurrent pain who comes from a painful family is most unlikely to grow up symptom-free.

Pupil Reactions

In Philadelphia, Rubin et al (1967) showed that, by measuring the reactions of the pupils, autonomic dysfunction can be demonstrated in children with recurrent abdominal pain. A previous Bristol report (Apley et al, 1970), confirmed the dysfunction, in general, and we have now completed a further and more detailed series. The two main points to come out in our series are, 1) in children with recurrent abdominal pain (or with asthma) the pupils tend to be larger than those of normal controls, both in the resting condition and under stress; 2) the change in pupil size with stress is less than in controls. Incidentally, an interesting new observation; a mother may occasionally have noticed that her child's pupils are enlarged with anxiety or perhaps with an attack of pain. What we do not know yet is whether the abnormal autonomic function is familial and inborn, though we are hoping to find out, and our preliminary study suggests that it is. Nor do we know if it is permanent or alterable. Should it prove to be inborn and permanent it will suggest that the expectations from treatment should not be set too high.

Treatment

I do not like the term 'informal psychotherapy': can you suggest a better one?*
The treatment we give is reassurance, based on explanations and discussions. 'No Reassurance without Explanation' (Apley & MacKeith, 1968). It cannot be claimed to have 'cured' the pains. It did effect a considerable difference by speeding the recovery from attacks of pain and, even more by lessening the occurrence of other symptoms both physical and nervous; it also increased the patient's adaptability and made it more likely that he could live a normal life.

In our follow-up of treated cases, half the patients were interviewed with their parents. The parents emphasised, time and again, the good effects of reassurance with explanations and discussions — on themselves as well as on the children.

As a result of some recent brilliant research work, I believe we should be able to do better still. I refer to Neil Miller's work which has revolutionised ideas on physiological responses (Miller, 1969). He has shown that autonomic responses can be modified by operant conditioning techniques, i.e. rewards which are given only when the appropriate autonomic response is elicited and can then modify the response. The method has been applied, by Miller and by others, to rats (to salivation, heart rate, intestinal activity, blood flow in the ear or in the kidney). Humans (including medical students) have been treated as successfully as have rats. Miller speculates that if a child experiences anxiety due to any cause, such as going to school, together with the autonomic symptoms with which we are familiar, the mother could reinforce one or more of the symptoms (e.g. abdominal pain) by drawing attention to it, making a fuss of the child and keeping him from school. I believe some doctors in practice do just this. Our job, surely, must be to find ways of rewarding the child *when he is well*. This, I guess, is the basis of *'No reassurance without explanations'.* It represents the clinical approach of doctors who are interested in the whole child rather than in giving drugs for a symptom.

References

Apley, J (1975) *The Child with Abdominal Pains, 2nd Edition.* Blackwell, Oxford
Apley, J, Haslam, D R and Tulloh, C G (1970) *Archives of Disease in Childhood, 46,* 337
Apley, J and MacKeith, R (1968) *The Child and his Symptoms. A Comprehensive approach, 2nd Edition.* Blackwell, Oxford.
Apley, J and Naish, N (1958) *Archives of Disease in Childhood, 33,* 165
Miller, N E (1969), *Science, 163,* 434
Rubin, L S, Barbero, G J, and Sibinga, M S (1967) *Psychosomatic Medicine, 29,* 111

*Professor Donald Court, in a note to me, suggests "informal personal doctoring".

Recurrent Abdominal Pain in Children
A Surgeon's Views

J LARI

A paediatric surgeon dealing with children with recurrent abdominal pain perhaps sees a more selected type of patient. The child with pain and other symptoms that may favour a functional cause is more likely to be referred to a paediatric physician.

I feel it is important to take a good *detailed history* and do a careful examination. This will save a lot of time later. It is vital to gain the confidence of the child and parent and show that you are genuinely interested in the problem and want to help. This is important because the child and his parent have often seen several doctors already and the attitude of the parent may be quite hostile at times.

It is usual for the *physical examination* to be quite normal and the history may give clues as to which *investigations* should be done. My normal practice is to do a urine examination, haemoglobin, white cell count and ESR. If the physical examination is negative and the investigations are normal, then with peri-umbilical pain and no other pointers, I may not do any X-ray examination, but ask to see the child during an attack and often do a straight film of the abdomen at that time. However, if the pain is to one or other side of the umbilicus, I ask for an intravenous pylogram and with epigastric pain, then a barium meal and follow through may be useful.

Like most clinicians I feel an intravenous pyelogram is more rewarding. If an anomaly is present it is more likely to cause irrevocable harm should it be missed. On the other hand, a delay in the diagnosis of a condition in the gastrointestinal tract causes no real harm.

Usually all investigations come back normal and I then make sure both the child and the parents know this and indicate that we have excluded any serious disease. It is important to make sure that the parents do not think that you are at any time suggesting that their child is not having genuine pain. At this point I quote Apley's (1975) findings on the incidence of recurrent abdominal pain in children and make them realise that this is a common problem and it is usual not to find any abnormality.

I do at times prescribe some *treatment* and I must own up to this. In some cases the pain is simply due to constipation and the symptoms improve if this is treated by simple means. Tranquillisers and sedatives I have no experience with and I do not believe they help. Antispasmodics like Merbentyl I have used in a selected few who have daily symptoms and it appears to help some, although Illingworth (1971) suggests that it is unhelpful. Antacids don't appear to work and from a study I did in these children there is no good reason why they should work.

Nineteen children who had recurrent abdominal pain with normal investigations, including a barium meal, had acid secretion studies in the form of a pentagastrin test. Table I shows the result. The children were between 5 and 14 years. Seven of these were girls. Comparing the peak acid output in these with children of the same age group with duodenal ulcers, we can see that they had lower secretions. For obvious ethical reasons we couldn't test children with no symptoms. However, when comparing them with normal adult volunteers who had the same test, we see that they match very well.

TABLE I. Peak Gastric Acid Secretions in Children and Adults

Group	Condition	Numbers	Mean peak secretion mEq/10 kg/hr
Children 5–14 years	Abdominal Pain	19 (7 girls)	4.43 (1.49–7.74)
	Duodenal ulcer.	13 (4 girls)	5.49 (3.74–9.10)
Adult Males 20–50 years	Normal	41	4.22
	Duodenal ulcer	80	6.80

So although this group of children tend to have more anxiety and come from families where there is an increased incidence of ulcers, in this small study their acid production appears to fall within the normal range.

I would like to mention two interesting children with recurrent abdominal pain seen recently. Both developed pain after drinking. Figure 1 explains the mechanism of their symptoms clearly. This is an intravenous pyelogram before and after the child took two glasses of water. The picture on the left is before the water-load and shows slight left-sided hydronephrosis and the one on the right shows a dramatic picture of hydronephrosis due to pelvi-uteri obstruction. This is not an uncommon symptom in adults with this condition but I have not seen it reported in children.

I feel that on this positive note, in this subject where there are a lot of negative findings, it is a good point to stop.

189

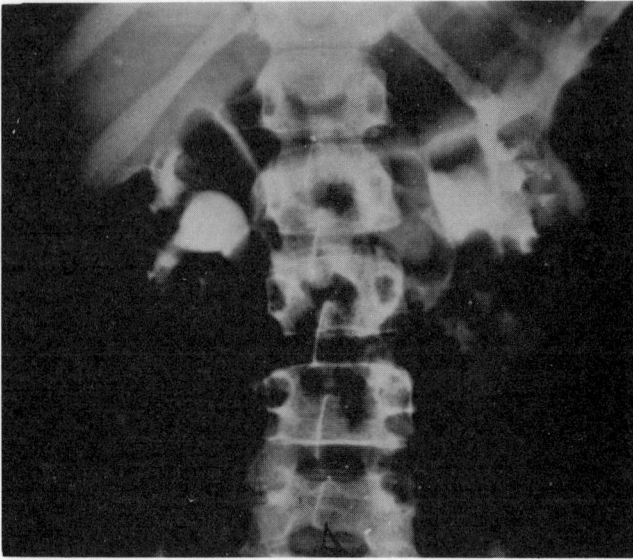

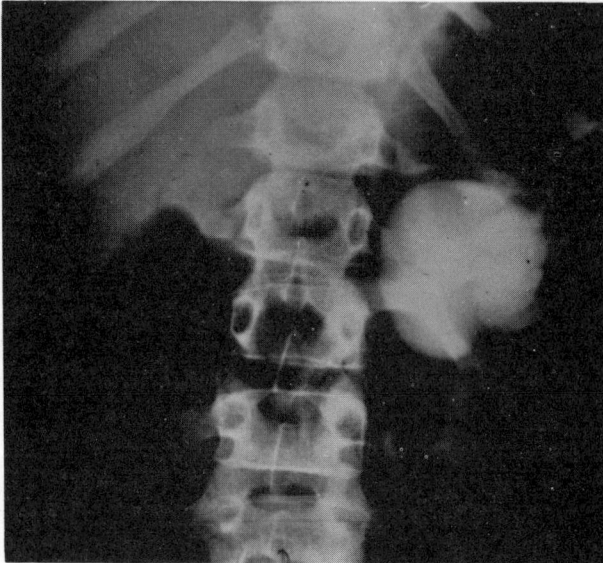

Figure 1. Intravenous pyelogram showing left-sided hydronephrosis. Before and after water-load.

References

Apley, J (1975) *The Child with Abdominal Pain. Second edition.* Blackwell Scientific Publications, Oxford

Illingworth, R S (1971) *The Treatment of the Child at Home.* Blackwell Scientific Publications, Oxford

Panel Discussion
ABDOMINAL PAIN

CHAIRMAN We've obviously covered an enormous range of things this after-
noon and while we ought not to structure the discussion to make it rigid perhaps we shouldn't allow Dr Apley to take us immediately to his eye-catching
95% of patients without organic diagnosis. I would like to ask the panel, then
the audience, what they feel is the proper investigational procedure in a child
who has recurring abdominal pain. Dr Dodge, you mentioned gastroscopy.
Would you like to begin?

DODGE Normally I think we have much the same policy as John Apley and
don't do much beyond a urine and blood count and perhaps an ESR and then
see them again in a month or so. I think that a great deal of information is got
from the history, that really these children with recurrent abdominal pain and
emotional problems are fairly characteristic in their presentation, and often
between the ages of 6 and 9 years. When the onset is older than that I think
one must look harder for an organic cause, and possibly, though I am not
quite so sure about this, in the younger age group as well. Recently we have
been doing gastroduodenoscopies, often at the request of colleagues, and on
occasion have found lesions we were not expecting. I think this may prove to
be a very useful method of investigating selected children.

CHAIRMAN Dr Apley, could you tell us what investigations of an organic
nature you do in your cases before deciding that you don't know what is
wrong with them?

APLEY It varies. For instance, in the last five years I have done a blood count
quite often, which I never did before. Why? Because someone showed that of
all the mothers whose children come up to any hospital, a quarter think they
have got leukaemia. So you have got to do a blood count. Similarly, the only
time I want to do a barium meal is to prove that there is *no* ulcer. If there *is*
an ulcer I don't want them to know. I think treatment is exactly the same as

if there is not. You are just labelling a child for the rest of his life. Barbero, in Philadelphia, and I sounded each other out terribly cautiously on this not so long ago; the moment a peptic ulcer is diagnosed radiologically, I would wait a week or so and get the X-rays repeated, often the ulcer is not there. Barbero does a routine second barium meal within 48 hours and most of the time it's not there. So what are we diagnosing?

DODGE   I can't really agree with John Apley about not telling patients when they have ulcers. I always tell them, and find that they are relieved that someone has at last made a diagnosis. That often does a great deal in itself by explaining the patient's symptoms and taking him seriously and showing that he's got a good reason to have a pain. I wouldn't keep this diagnosis to myself because I think the patient has a right to know, the parents have a right to know, and they have a right to some sort of management for it even though the treatment may not be very successful.

APLEY   I agree you can't keep it secret. That's why you shouldn't do a barium meal.

ROSSITER   Do you think there is any relationship between recurrent abdominal pain in childhood and irritable bowel syndrome in adults? Either in common aetiology or one turning into the other?

APLEY   I don't like the diagnosis of 'irritable colon' at all. I think the *patient* is irritable and therefore it shows in one or other part of him, and it happens to be in the gut.

CHAIRMAN   Perhaps you could come in here, Dr Morris. You mentioned irritable bowels, and also the 50% of your adults with abdominal pain you didn't know what was wrong with.

MORRIS   I think there was a report from one of the Scandinavian countries, in which they did a follow-up of children who had recurrent abdominal pain and showed that a proportion of them had peptic ulcers, irritable bowel, and diverticular disease in adult life. I thought that was very relevant information. Certainly looking at it at the other end of the life span, one does get a history of abdominal pain occurring in bouts in childhood, in patients whom one thinks has an irritable bowel syndrome. I think Dr Apley is maligning the gastroenterologist a little in saying it doesn't exist because there is reasonable physiological evidence to show that bouts of abdominal pain in patients who have this syndrome coincide with high pressure zones within the gastrointestinal tract. Dr Heaton is in the audience, I am sure he can tell us that administering fibre or similar preparation to patients with irritable bowel syndrome can often abolish their pain and, what is more significant perhaps, lower resting intracolonic pressures which seems to me to mean that there is a pathological process going on within the bowel of patients with an irritable bowel.

McNEISH   Dr Heaton, are you prepared to support him?

HEATON   I'm certainly prepared to support him to the extent of believing that there is an entity which we call irritable bowel syndrome and of course very often there are changes in bowel habit coinciding with episodic pain, even though it is not clear where the pain is coming from. You can reproduce the pain by blowing air up through a sigmoidoscope and that sort of thing. I agree that one's experience is that many of them are relieved by the diet but I know also that the treatment has a tremendous placebo effect.

CHAIRMAN   You must also see many adults with abdominal pain, and you don't know what the cause is. Is there a relation between that and the irritable bowel syndrome? Do bellyaching adults have an irritable bowel?

HEATON   Yes, I think so. I found that when you take a more detailed bowel history, you will find that there are certain changes in bowel habit in many people with functional dyspepsia.

CHAIRMAN   Your children, John, do they have irritable bowels?

APLEY   Well, you see, the worry is that on the whole they talk about some relation with eating or defaecation, colic and pellet stools and so on. I don't find these in little babies and children. I may be wrong. A lot of them keep going to the lavatory.

WALKER-SMITH   We sometimes see children with Crohn's disease, which is more common in the older child, over the age of 10. Sometimes those children do have a history of long-term pain blending into this syndrome, and I think doing an ESR may be something that's useful. I have seen 3 or 4 children with advanced Crohn's disease who have had abdominal pain, though I realise that's very rare.

WEAVER   I wonder if Dr Apley would agree that there is a small group of children who readily become ketotic for one reason or another who present with vomiting and abdominal pain?

APLEY   Sure, but I don't think it's a cause. It's part of an upset and if you smell the breath of any child who comes into hospital a large proportion of them are ketotic.

CHAIRMAN   Dr Pinkerton, we invited you on to the platform, we haven't heard your views. Dr Apley has made the point that the sort of patients we see are maybe the ones we are interested in so I would guess that you might also have a selected population. Perhaps you would like to comment on the presentation, and on the numbers of *your* patients that have organic disorders, first of all?

PINKERTON   I'm in the very fortunate position of having a built-in filter because I work in the biggest children's hospital in the British Commonwealth. Therefore all my patients come through my paediatric, or paediatric surgical, colleagues. If it's an organic lesion that is missed, I am not missing it, which is a very happy position to be in. Which brings me to the point that I never diagnose functional disorder, unless I can demonstrate convincingly to my colleagues or the parents of the patient and to myself positive evidence in support of it being functional. I never ever make a diagnosis of functional disorder on a negative basis, because I believe it's a very dangerous thing to do. You must take a careful enough history. The story must be convincing enough to you to explain the symptoms in terms of emotional disturbance.

MELVILLE-THOMAS   I would like to ask, on that point, how many paediatricians take a separate history from the child and from the parent? Maybe it ought to be a sort of double-barrelled one, one from the child and one from the parents, and maybe we would get a different picture.

SIBERT   One sees quite a lot of girls, in adolescence, who have reached puberty, but not yet reached the menarche, who come in with abdominal pain. Do you think these pains are purely due to emotional causes or do you think there might be physiological reasons?

PINKERTON   I'll deal with this quickly, because in a recent paper it was said that the onset of abdominal pain is highest in girls at the age of 9 and then it gets less. It must be too early for puberty.

CHAIRMAN   Professor Hadorn, in your view, is this a British condition we are looking at?

HADORN   It is very frequent also in our country. There is one little point I would like to comment upon. One of our surgeons, Professor Beckte, used to say that even repeated urinary examination for leucocytes in the urine were not sufficient to exclude the presence of malformation and so we are rather liberal with doing an intravenous pyelogram in these children if there really is a recurrence of the symptoms.

CHAIRMAN   Perhaps now we could talk about treatment or indeed anything else that you want. Are there any other points?

QUESTION FROM AUDIENCE   I'd like to ask Dr Sibert about this question of the spuriously high serum amylase. As you say, it can come about as the result of increased levels of binding protein. Can I ask first of all has the protein, the nature of the protein, been identified? Then, if that is so, perhaps the normal levels that one is getting in children who one suspects have pancreatitis may be due simply to a low level of the protein.

SIBERT   First of all, I think macroamylasaemia is a poorly understood condition, and probably many different conditions produce this spuriously high amylase. I do not think that people are missing many cases of acute pancreatitis in children. I think it must be a very rare syndrome. Having said that, doing the amylase during the acute attack of abdominal pain is not a bad investigation to do, because blood is going to be taken anyway at that time and it is not going to involve the child in any undue discomfort. I don't think it is worth while doing it in Out-Patients, unless it is during an attack of pain.

NELSON   Dr Apley mentioned the importance of control groups in this sort of situation. He mentioned the emotional factors and the personality factors, but there are large numbers of children who have similar emotional problems or similar personality factors who do not get abdominal pain. Have the investigations of the emotional and personality side of this situation been as well controlled as the EEG examination, IVPs etc?

APLEY   That's a good point. I'm no psychiatrist. You learn from your colleagues and I think one of the most important things we have to learn in paediatrics is to listen to psychiatrists and psychiatric social workers. We checked our own results in two or three ways. We took a school series and a hospital series. A child psychiatrist examined the hospital series as we did, without our knowledge, and got very similar figures. We then compared them with the school children and they were almost the same. I can't say I've gone in for personality tests.

CHAIRMAN   Dr Pinkerton? Would you like to come in on that?

PINKERTON   I think I would say that there is a factor in these cases which I always regard as highly suspect, but if there is a family history of this type coupled with a particular type of personality, that's very suggestive. John Apley mentioned a *symptom choice,* which is a very fascinating area. When there isn't a history of this kind in the family, you are on very much shakier ground and I am sure there has not been any evidence so far to convincingly demonstrate why someone should choose one system and some choose another. Very many years ago someone came out with an aphorism that, vhereas the seat of adult malaise is the head, the seat of malaise for children

195

is the 'tummy'. If you ask children 'Where do you feel funny?', they will more often point to their tummies than anywhere else and I think this is a useful thing to demonstrate.

HARRIES   I wonder if I could ask the panel how many children do you think who say that they have a 'tummy-ache' don't actually *have* the tummy-ache, but use the word in a different context, with a different meaning.

APLEY   I would say that the experienced clinician isn't very easily foxed about whether there is in children an abdominal origin or there isn't. I don't think you miss many acute organic disorders, whatever the child tells you. You have to draw the line somewhere, and we do not include in our studies any child who has not had at least three bouts which should have affected their play or work. In addition, a large proportion of them go pale and lie down, so I think with those that we have included, the pain is just as real as any other pain.

CHAIRMAN   We have had trouble with this 'autonomic dysfunctional reactivity' we were talking about. Dr Apley, tell me how you do pupilometry.

APLEY   We put the child's hand in ice cold water for 5 seconds and see what happens to his pupils. We have found that in these children the pupil was too big and under stress did not react enough.

WALKER-SMITH   I have been impressed when doing out-patient clinics just how frequent a family history of migraine really is. I think that a lot of the abdominal pain that I have seen may be related to what was described as abdominal migraine, if by that one might mean that some form of vascular instability, is related to more widespread vascular disturbance than just the head. I wonder what the panel think of that, but might I just couple that remark with another question? A few years ago a paper described a series of young people with what was called hypertrophic duodenitis. These individuals were X-rayed and they did not have duodenal ulcers. Have you seen this syndrome? Has it been diagnosed by endoscopy? How do we treat it?

MORRIS   It was published about 7 years ago and the authors described hypertrophic duodenitis with a very high acid secretion (Rhodes, Evans, Lawrie & Forrest, 1968). I think this is a very rare syndrome. It is possible of course that you can have a pre-peptic ulcer condition.

DODGE   I think there is no doubt that you get duodenal ulcer symptoms without ulceration. You can have an inflamed haemorrhagic duodenal mucosa where perhaps because of a technical inadequacy, we don't actually see a crater. Quite obviously there must be a stage at which the mucosa is inflamed before you get a hole in it, and after it has healed when it may still be a little bit inflamed, but I would agree with you that this entity of hypertrophic duodenitis seems to be rare.

MORRIS   May I just come back on that one point? I would suspect that this is called duodenitis and is described as 'pepper and salt ulcerations' in the duodenum. I really do think that every time we diagnose this condition we make a rod for our own backs, because there is nothing we can do about it. Indeed, the work from Birmingham which was recently published has shown that if you do vagotomies on these patients, you are in fact doing them a great disservice.

LARI   I would expect to see an ulcer or duodenitis after a pyloromyotomy, if they have had an incomplete vagotomy perhaps, or even in the ones who have had an exploration.

Can I come to what John was saying earlier about duodenal ulcers in children who have pyloromyotomy? I am wondering, although perhaps I shouldn't say it to this audience, whether in fact the surgery is causing some problems of co-ordination of the muscle of the pylorus, and therefore it is the surgeon who is later on giving the children ulcers, rather than the original pyloric stenosis.

DODGE   I think you are actually maligning your own branch of the profession, because there is some evidence, although it is not terribly well controlled, that there is an increased incidence of peptic ulceration in the *relatives* of children with pyloric stenosis, who have never had Ramstedt's operation, so that presumably there is therefore a familial ulcer tendency.

If I can come from that to John Apley and John Morris, I wonder if between them they can work out for us the sort of pathway or mechanism by which children with 'belly-ache' due to emotional causes actually get it. Why do they get a pain? How does it arise? What do you think actually happens?

MORRIS   I think that Dr Apley's suggestion about heightened sensitivity is a very attractive one but perhaps one should look for more precise physiological evidence although that would be very difficult to obtain. One would have to look for various autonomic reflexes such as looking for pupil changes after dipping hands into cold water, responses to adrenaline or nor-adrenaline, which I think might be relevant to the problem.

On the other hand we all have intestinal gas and it might be that if you have a heightened sensitivity in the autonomic nervous system, that gas, which is normally present in everybody, causes more problems.

APLEY   I have always suspected a vascular shift. That is, blood goes from the skin, which gets white to the gut which gets red, only I didn't know how to set about investigating it. Barbero looks inside the rectum and he says there is a difference in the depth of colour.

HARRIES   I was wondering whether Dr Apley believed in the work of Davidson about 10 years ago, who undertook motility studies on his children and found pressure changes. Do you think this plays any part?

APLEY   I don't think it does, John. I think it is only an expression of the total change so that if the patient is irritable, the moment you stick a label on one bit or part, I think you have done a disservice to the whole self.

HADORN   Dr Apley, you spoke of results and what you tell the parents. Are these the results of an attitude, or are these the results of something you have told the parents?

APLEY   Very briefly, we can't cure anybody's pains but I think we can make them less; we can make them less likely to occur. We can certainly stop patients getting more nervous and psychosomatic syndromes than if we just ignore them. When we went round these families twelve or fifteen years later to ask how they had got on, they said the moment somebody explained, they were so relieved, and they were then able to live with the symptoms. Our figures show they lead normal lives now although the pain still comes back.

Reference
Rhodes J, Evans K T , Lawrie J H & Forrest A P M; 1968. *Quarterly Journal of Medicine*, Volume *145*, pages 151–169

Constipation

The Pathophysiology of Constipation in Children

E R HOWARD

Constipation may present in many ways and it is difficult to give a definition of the condition which will encompass all of the clinical symptoms and signs. Definitions may be based, for example, on whether the colon or the rectum is the portion of gut most affected, or on the number of bowel actions per week, or on the time taken for the transit of ingested material through the gastrointestinal tract. In the present discussion constipation is defined as infrequent defaecation which is accomplished with some difficulty. The motions are usually hard and the rectum is not emptied completely. It is accepted that this description excludes many symptoms which are rather more variable in occurrence, such as malaise, abdominal distension, and abdominal pain. This review is concerned with the classification, physiology and morphology of constipation.

AETIOLOGICAL CLASSIFICATION

The causes of constipation may be classified in many ways (Table I). Efficient emptying of the bowel, however, is achieved by co-ordinated contractions of the hindgut which depend on the integrity of nervous plexuses within the bowel wall. The important causes of constipation have therefore been grouped according to the presence or absence of normal ganglia within the gut.

TABLE I. Causes of Constipation

NORMAL GANGLIA			ABNORMAL GANGLIA
Intrinsic	Extrinsic	Functional	Aganglionosis
Abnormal faeces	Birth stress	Simple constipation	Hypoganglionosis
Anatomical malformations	Spinal cord lesions	Megacolon	Neurofibromatosis
Tumours	Metabolic abnormalities	Megarectum	Chagas disease Laxatives
			Cytotoxic agents Lipidoses

Normal Ganglia Present

Difficult defaecation may be caused by *intrinsic* abnormalities such as anatomical malformations or increased viscosity of faeces. Anatomical anomalies affecting the ano-rectum are mostly obvious from birth (Stephens & Durham Smith, 1971) although congenital anal stenosis may be missed at first (Harris et al, 1954). An increase in the viscosity of faeces is seen at its extreme in approximately 10% of newborn infants with fibrocystic disease when the meconium is viscid enough to cause complete intestinal obstruction. Long plugs of meconium with an increased stickiness possibly caused by an excessive reabsorption of water (Emery, 1957) may obstruct the colon in the unrelated meconium-plug syndrome of the newborn (Clatworthy et al, 1956; Mikity et al, 1967).

Abnormalities *extrinsic* to the gut wall, which include lesions of the central nervous system and general metabolic diseases, may affect bowel activity. A variable degree of bowel dysfunction in the stressed newborn infant is not uncommon (MacLaurin, 1964) and the many factors that have been incriminated in its causation include anoxia, cerebral birth trauma, dehydration, rhesus incompatibility and exsanguination (Dunn, 1963), ganglion blocking agents for the treatment of maternal hypertension (Morris, 1953; Hallum & Hatchuel, 1954) and maternal heroin addiction (Raffensperger et al, 1961). Metabolic states associated with depressed bowel motility include hypothyroidism, hypercalcaemia from the ingestion of excessive vitamin D (Henderson, 1968) and porphyria (Goodall, 1967). Normal bowel evacuation is controlled and co-ordinated by a complex interplay of voluntary and autonomic nervous mechanisms which involve cerebral, spinal and peripheral nervous pathways. An absence of these pathways, for example in some children with myelomeningocele or neoplasm of the spinal canal, may cause constipation even when normal ganglia are present within the bowel wall.

A majority of children with constipation do not have a detectable cause for their symptoms and are described as having a *'functional'* abnormality. Histological examination of the bowel wall is unremarkable and the peripheral nervous pathways are intact. The children may present with constipation at any age but most commonly between 3 years and 9 years. A megacolon or megarectum may or may not develop. 'Functional' constipation may be evident from early infancy and this has been cited as evidence for a genetic factor (Coekin & Gairdner, 1960). After a study of twins, Bakwin and Davidson (1971) reported that monozygotic pairs were concordant for constipation nearly four times as frequently as were dizygotic twins. Significant parent-child concordance for constipation was also noted in this study. The authors concluded that the genetic predisposition to constipation is expressed by both excessive water absorption and increased rectal muscular tone with the consequent production of small firm stools. A relationship has also been reported between personality and bowel disorders which include constipation (Jost & Sontog, 1944).

201

Little is known about the development of a normal bowel habit (Bentley, 1971). It is not known, for example, how colonic evacuation is inhibited in utero although 94% of normal infants pass meconium within the first 24 hours of birth (Sherry & Kramer, 1955). In the infant large bowel contractions are stimulated by sucking and feeding so that defaecation is frequent during the first few months of life. As development proceeds the frequency of bowel actions is reduced. This process is helped by a combination of factors which include the introduction of a more solid, mixed diet and the inhibition by the central nervous system of colo-rectal reflexes which is developed through training and social taboos. By three years of age the child learns to pass faeces once or twice per day and, perhaps more importantly, in a socially acceptable place (Brazelton, 1962). Disturbances in behaviour patterns at this time can easily be reflected in disturbances of bowel physiology which may present as either incontinence (encopresis) or as faecal retention with or without faecal overflow (Oppé, 1967). The causation of a painful anal fissure by large or hard stools exacerbates the problem by inducing a further suppression of reflex responses, and rectal sensation may be lost by chronic stretching of the rectal wall (Nixon, 1967).

Abnormal Ganglia

Congenital, infective and drug-induced abnormalities of inter-muscular and sub-mucosal ganglia have now been identified. These abnormalities cause disordered contraction and relaxation of the bowel musculature and a consequent loss of efficient bowel evacuation which may range from simple constipation to complete obstruction. These conditions will be discussed individually in the section on morphological observations.

PHYSIOLOGICAL INVESTIGATIONS

Physiological methods of investigating constipation include the use of barium in conventional and cine-radiography, transit-time markers, colonic manometry, ano-rectal manometry and electromyography of the pelvic floor. Clinically these investigations can be used (1) to decide whether the patient is truly constipated; (2) to measure the severity of secondary changes that may have occurred in the bowel wall, and (3) to assess the response to treatment.

Barium studies may be necessary to exclude an intrinsic mechanical cause for constipation and are diagnostic for congenital aganglionosis (Bodian et al, 1949). They are also useful for assessing the size of a megacolon or megarectum. Barium can also be used as a marker of intestinal transit-time (Shanks & Kerley, 1958), although it may become inspissated in the large bowel and require vigorous treatment for evacuation. Hurst (1919) used charcoal as a transit-marker and defined constipation as a 'condition in which none of the residue of a meal taken 8 hours after defaecation is excreted within 40 hours'. Other markers that have been used include beads (Alvarez & Freelander, 1924), carmine (Dimson, 1970), radio-opaque pellets (Hinton & Lennard-Jones, 1968), and radio-isotopically labelled substances such as C^{14}-polyethylene glycol (Wingate et al, 1972; Smith, 1973). Dimson (1970) showed that a dose of 0.3 g of carmine was usually excreted by the fourth day after ingestion in children with normal bowel habits whereas in 60 out of 65 constipated children the time interval was extended to between 5 and 13 days after ingestion. Similarly Hinton and Lennard-Jones (1968) found that the excretion of radio-opaque pellets commenced within 72 hours of ingestion in all of 25 asymptomatic adults.

Measures of colonic motility have been made from recordings of colonic intraluminal pressures (Davidson et al, 1956). Although these techniques are too time-consuming for routine clinical use they do show typical patterns of activity in constipated individuals. Connell (1962), for example, has described the paradoxically *increased* segmental activity of the colon in constipation. Constipated patients who have received an injection of prostigmine also show an absence of the normal decreasing gradient of activity from sigmoid colon to rectum (Waller & Misiewicz, 1972).

The ano-rectum is more easily accessible to physiological investigation than the colon and the synchronous recording of rectal pressures with the mechanical and electrical activity of the anal sphincters is helpful in the investigation and management of constipation. Simplified techniques for making these recordings in clinical practice have been described by Schuster (1965) and Lawson and Nixon (1967). Both techniques include devices for inflating the rectum so that measures of rectal capacity and sensation can be taken at the same time as recordings of reflex activity between the rectum and internal and external anal sphincters. Distension of a normal rectum with a bolus of air or fluid causes a rectal contraction and a sensation of rectal fullness referred to the sacro-perineal region. The rectal contraction is accompanied by a relaxation of the smooth muscle of the internal sphincter and a contraction of the voluntary muscle of the external sphincter which ensures continence. At a critical level of rectal distension the voluntary sphincter is also inhibited and defaecation results (Howard, 1969).

Specific abnormalities are seen in recordings taken from patients with Hirschsprung's disease. The aganglionic rectum exhibits repeated contractions of variable duration and amplitude which are accentuated by rectal distension. An absence of reflex relaxation of the internal anal sphincter provides the basis of a clinical screening test for aganglionosis (Howard, 1972).

Characteristic changes of ano-rectal physiology may also be recorded from patients with 'functional' constipation. Callaghan and Nixon (1964) divided the severity of the rectal changes into 3 grades: (1) *the enlarged rectum* − a larger distending volume than normal is needed to produce inhibition of the anal sphincters; (2) *the expanded rectum* − rectal pressure changes occur only after a loading

203

volume of air; (3) *the inert rectum* — a large distending volume is necessary in the rectum to cause inhibition of the sphincters which eventually occurs without rectal sensation. This situation is found in patients with faecal soiling.

The severity of rectal changes in chronic constipation may therefore be graded and the effectiveness of any treatment assessed by repeated physiological examination.

The observation that anal sphincter relaxation may be poor in some constipated children until the rectum is maximally distended led Lawson (1974) to examine the effects of anal stretch on constipation. Forty-two per cent of a group of 46 children who underwent anal stretching were completely cured and a further 38% showed some improvement.

Temporary abnormalities of ano-rectal physiology have been reported in stressed newborn infants with intestinal obstruction in whom no mechanical cause was found and from whom ganglionic gut biopsies were obtained (Howard & Nixon, 1968). Physiological responses became normal during the following 2—3 weeks as symptoms subsided.

MORPHOLOGICAL OBSERVATIONS

Abnormalities in the intrinsic innervation of the bowel have been identified in some children with constipation and explain the disordered physiology in these patients.

Congenital Aganglionosis (Hirschsprung's Disease)

This was well documented as 'congenital megacolon' for at least 70 years before the nervous lesion was identified (Whitehouse & Kernohan, 1948; Zuelzer & Wilson, 1948; Bodian et al, 1949). All of these reports described an absence of ganglion cells in variable lengths of rectum and colon, the aganglionosis always starting, however, at the anal canal and extending in a cranial direction. Most reported cases of aganglionosis have shown this distribution of affected bowel but more recently MacIver and Whitehead (1972) described zonal *colonic* aganglionosis in 4 out of 15 cases of Hirschsprung's disease and collected 7 further cases from the literature. Histochemical studies have revealed a more complex abnormality in Hirschsprung's disease than a simple absence of ganglion cells and this has helped to explain the variability in the severity of symptoms in different patients with similar lengths of aganglionic bowel. The absence of ganglion cells is only part of a defect which includes an abnormal distribution of nerves for some distance above the aganglionic zone. In addition there is a marked variation in the number of acetylcholinesterase-positive nerves in the circular muscle and a very abnormal distribution of adrenergic nerves (Garrett et al, 1969; Howard, 1972).

204

Smith (1975) has recently found a reduced number of ganglia in colons resected from 5 patients with idiopathic megacolon which suggests a condition of *congenital hypoganglionosis.* Similarly Bentley (1964) described a zone of hypoganglionosis just proximal to the internal anal sphincter in 5 constipated children treated by anal-myotomy. This zone is difficult to assess histologically, however, as a zone of hypoganglionosis may extend from 2 to 4 cm above the mucocutaneous junction of the anal canal in the normal individual (Hofmann & Orestano, 1967; Aldridge & Campbell, 1969).

Plexiform neurofibromatosis

Affecting the myenteric plexus as well as other parts of the body this may present with symptoms and X-ray changes remarkably similar to congenital aganglionosis (Staple et al, 1964; Ternberg & Winters, 1965).

Chagas' disease

Endemic in South America, this is of interest in this discussion as it demonstrates the effects of a progressive loss of enteric ganglia on bowel motility (Köberle, 1963). Ganglionic neurones are destroyed by a neurotoxin of the parasite *Trypanosoma cruzi* which is transmitted to man by the Reduviid bug. The patient may develop megaoesophagus and conduction defects in the heart as well as severe constipation and megacolon. There is a loss of peristalsis and the bowel becomes dilated down to the pelvic floor.

The long-term use of laxatives – particularly those of the anthraquinone group such as senna and cascara – may cause irreversible damage to the nerve plexuses of the bowel wall. Smith (1968) has described fragmentation of axons and the development of axonal and dendritic swellings after the use of these drugs. The colon loses its contractile activity and its haustral pattern and may eventually develop into a thin-walled megacolon: the *cathartic colon.*

Cytotoxic agents may affect the intrinsic nervous system of the bowel. Vincristine and vinblastine, for example, which are used in a variety of malignant diseases, may affect the autonomic nervous system through their action on neurotubules (Wisneiwski et al, 1968). The brain is protected by the blood-brain barrier but Smith (1972) has described extensive damage to nerves in the bowel wall in patients who have received vincristine before death. Clinically, dilatation of the large and small bowel may occur with constipation. Other drugs which may affect the bowel include chlorpromazine (Zimmerman, 1962), mepacrine (Keeler et al, 1966), isonicotinic acid hydrazide (Smith, 1967), and amitriptyline (Burkitt & Sutcliffe, 1961; Gander & Devlin, 1963).

References

Aldridge, R T and Campbell, P E (1968) *Journal of Pediatric Surgery, 3,* 475
Alvarez, W C and Freedlander, B L (1924) *Journal of the American Medical Association, 83,* 576
Bakwin, H and Davidson, M (1971) *American Journal of Diseases of Children, 121,* 179
Bentley, J F R (1964) *Diseases of the Colon and Rectum, 7,* 462
Bentley, J F R (1971) *Gut, 12,* 85
Bodian, M, Stephens, F D and Ward, B C H (1949) *Lancet, 1,* 6
Brazelton, T B (1962) *Pediatrics, 29,* 121
Burkitt, E A and Sutcliffe, C K (1961) *British Medical Journal, 2,* 1648
Callaghan, R P and Nixon, H H (1964) *Archives of Disease in Childhood, 39,* 153
Clatworthy, H W, Howard, W H R and Lloyd, J (1956) *Surgery, 39,* 131
Coekin, M and Gairdner, D (1960) *British Medical Journal, 2,* 1175
Connell, A M (1962) *Gut, 3,* 342
Davidson, M, Sleisenger, M H, Almy, T P and Levine, S Z (1956) *Pediatrics, 17,* 807
Dimson, S B (1970) *Archives of Disease in Childhood, 45,* 232
Dunn, P (1963) *Archives of Disease in Childhood, 38,* 459
Emery, J (1957) *Archives of Disease in Childhood, 32,* 17
Gander, D R and Devlin, H B (1963) *British Medical Journal, 1,* 1160
Garrett, J R, Howard, E R and Nixon, H H (1969) *Archives of Disease in Childhood, 44,* 406
Goodall, J (1967) *Proceedings of the Royal Society of Medicine, 60,* 1001
Hallum, J L and Hatchuel, W L F (1954) *Archives of Disease in Childhood, 29,* 354
Harris, L E, Corbin, H P F and Hill, J R (1954) *Pediatrics, 13,* 59
Henderson, W (1968) *Postgraduate Medical Journal, 44,* 724
Hinton, J M and Lennard-Jones, J E (1968) *Postgraduate Medical Journal, 44,* 720
Hofmann, S and Orestano, F (1967) *Journal of Pediatric Surgery, 2,* 575
Howard, E R (1969) In *Recent Advances in Paediatric Surgery, 2nd Edition* (Ed.) A W Wilkinson. Churchill, London. Pages 77–87
Howard, E R (1972) *Postgraduate Medical Journal, 48,* 471
Howard, E R and Nixon, H H (1968) *Archives of Disease in Childhood, 43,* 569
Hurst, A F (1919) In *Constipation and Allied Intestinal Disorders, 2nd Edition,* Oxford Medical Publications, London. Page 55
Jost, H and Sontog, L W (1944) *Psychosomatic Medicine, 6,* 308
Keeler, R, Richardson, H and Watson, A J (1966) *Laboratory Investigations, 15,* 1253
Köberle, F (1963) *Gut, 4,* 399
Lawson, J O N (1974) *Archives of Disease in Childhood, 49,* 245
Lawson, J O N and Nixon, H H (1967) *Journal of Pediatric Surgery, 2,* 544
MacIver, A G and Whitehead, R (1972) *Archives of Disease in Childhood, 47,* 233
MacLaurin, C (1964) *Australian & New Zealand Journal of Surgery, 34,* 196
Morris, N (1953) *Lancet, 1,* 322
Nixon, H H (1967) *Proceedings of the Royal Society of Medicine, 60,* 801
Oppé, T E (1967) *Proceedings of the Royal Society of Medicine, 60,* 803
Raffensperger, J, Johnson, F R and Greengard, J (1961) *Surgery, 49,* 696
Schuster, M M, Hookman, P, Hendrix, T R and Mendeloff, A I (1965) *Johns Hopkins Hospital Bulletin, 116,* 79
Shanks, S C and Kerley, P (1958) In *A Textbook of X-ray Diagnosis,* vol. 3, 3rd Edition, Lewis, London. Page 367
Sherry, S N and Kramer, I (1955) *Journal of Pediatrics, 46,* 158
Smith, B (1967) *Journal of Neurology, Neurosurgery and Psychiatry, 30,* 506
Smith, B (1968) *Gut, 9,* 139
Smith, B (1972) In *The Neuropathology of the Alimentary Tract.* Arnold, London, Page 85
Smith, B (1975) in preparation
Smith, C L (1973) In *Fourth International Symposium on Gastrointestinal Motility* (Ed.) E E Daniel. Mitchell Press, Vancouver. Pages 353–354

Staple, T W, McAlister, W H and Anderson, M S (1964) *American Journal of Roentgenology, Radium Therapy and Nuclear Medicine, 91*, 840

Stephens, F D and Durham Smith, E (1971) *Ano-Rectal Malformations in Children*. Year Book Medical Publishers, Chicago.

Swenson, O, Sherman, J O and Fisher, J H (1973) *Journal of Pediatric Surgery, 8*, 587

Ternberg, J L and Winters, K (1965) *American Journal of Surgery, 109*, 663

Waller, S L and Misiewicz, J J (1972) *Scandinavian Journal of Gastroenterology, 7*, 93

Whitehouse, F R and Kernohan, J W (1948) *Archives of Internal Medicine, 82*, 75

Wingate, D L, Sandberg, R J and Phillips, S F (1972) *Gut, 13*, 812

Wisniewski, H, Shelanski, M L and Terry, R D (1968) *Journal of Cell Biology, 38*, 224

Zimmerman, G R (1962) *Archives of Pathology, 74*, 47

Zuelzer, W W and Wilson, J L (1948) *American Journal of Diseases of Children, 75*, 40

Psychological Factors in Childhood Constipation

PHILIP PINKERTON

Accuracy of Definition

If what is meant by constipation is sluggishness of bowel action, the most logical contribution to its development by any mental mechanism would be endogenous depression. This is a psycho-physiological sequence. In practice, however, true depression is rare in childhood, and in any case, hardly ever presents in the classical adult form of psychomotor retardation affecting peristalsis.

If, on the other hand, the American term 'obstipation' is adopted, this more typically reflects the mechanism in early childhood through which emotional factors characteristically affect bowel action. The aetiological clue lies in condensing the two words 'obstinate constipation' to emphasise the key factor of obstinate behaviour which motivates the syndrome.

Alternative Causal Factors

Other situations undoubtedly contribute to emotionally based constipation. They include faulty bowel training in infancy by feckless, inadequate or disorganised parents. If this persists, it leads in time to faulty bowel habit with resulting physiological sluggishness.

Alternatively, sudden frights associated with defaecation may inadvertently upset the toddler and thereby jeopardise recently acquired bowel control. There may be fantasies of being sucked down the toilet bowl especially when the flushing action is loud. Sometimes fears can be traced to careless adult comment about flushing undesirable things down the toilet which is then misinterpreted by the eavesdropping child. However, this kind of phobia, while it might precipitate transient reluctance to use the toilet, should not lead in itself to more persistent difficulties. If the problem is chronic, it is almost certainly being sustained by other factors.

Socio-economic circumstances may also contribute to problems in toilet training. There may be reluctance for example to use an outside toilet, especially after dark in winter time, and yet this may be the only facility available to the child other than the pot or bucket which he may feel he has outgrown.

208

Yet another contributory factor is persisting fear of painful defaecation after the original experience of an anal crack or small fissure. It is interesting in these circumstances to speculate upon what caused the fissure to develop originally!

Bowel Negativism

Nevertheless, although such diverse situations do present, the *classical* sequence in early childhood activating bowel dysfunction in emotional terms is undoubtedly *negativism*.

Age of Peak Incidence – the Toddler

During the first 18 months of life, development is dominated by progressive unfolding of the child's potential capacities. The hallmark of this phase is compliance or passivity in that the child remains largely dependent upon his mother in particular to gratify his essential needs.

Towards the end of this period, however, there is increasing self-awareness as a separate organism, and with that sense of independence there emerges the drive towards self-assertion. Increasingly as he learns to fend for himself – to articulate his needs verbally, to actively explore his environment, to attend to his own feeding, elimination etc. – so there is the tendency to become contrary about parental authority. This, it should be emphasised, is a perfectly normal phase of development. If handled wisely, it will gradually fade as the child matures and finds his own niche within the family (Pinkerton, 1974).

However, should undue emphasis be laid upon certain schedules, e.g. feeding routine, pattern of elimination, or bedtime routine, i.e. should parents attempt too rigidly to establish a rhythm of feeding, elimination or sleep, the toddler will sense it and his tendency to be defiant will almost certainly be channelled into that particular sphere. Henceforth battle will be joined over the issue of bed-time, feeding schedules, suitable diet, or, by the same token, bowel routine (Table I).

Of these various issues, the 'battle of the bowels' is one of the most difficult to resolve once the gauntlet has been thrown down. It is wise to bear in mind that it takes two or more to create a conflict.

Personality Profile

Negativism in the toddler is virtually a universal phenomenon. Nevertheless some children are more self-willed than others and evidence exists that individual differences can be identified in make-up as early as the first few months of life (Thomas et al, 1968). It is important therefore in this age group to take cognisance of the determined personality. Spontaneous comments by parents such as 'he's got a real will of his own' or 'when he digs his heels in, etc', can prove valuable diagnostic pointers and should never be ignored.

TABLE I. Stages of Emotional Development

	Infant	Toddler
Age Range	0–18 months	18 months – 3 years
Hallmark	Compliance	Defiance
Developmental characteristics	Maturation of potential capacities ↓ Social moulding by parental training	Awareness of self ↓ Independence from mother ↓ Self-assertion
Diagnostic patterns	Passive reflection of parental stress	Active negativism over ↓ Feeding Sleep Elimination

Modified from: *Childhood Disorder – A Psychosomatic Approach,* Philip Pinkerton. Published by Crosby Lockwood Staples, London. 1974.

Complementary Parental Profile

Winnicott (1958) claimed that there is no such thing as a baby. By this he meant to emphasise the baby's inability to survive on its own. The same holds true for emotional interaction. However defiant the toddler, his contrariness is unlikely to persist unless reinforced and thereby potentiated by complementary determination in the parent. When this happens, and the issue is focused on bowel function, the scene is set for the immovable mass (of inspissated faeces) to be met by the irresistable force (of parental coercion). This is one issue which the parent cannot hope to win. He may successfully overcome the child's resistance to defaecation by mechanical means such as repeated enemata, or by pharmaceutical agents such as powerful purgatives, but what he cannot command is the child's defaecation at the appropriate time and in the appropriate place.

Two main motivating factors are responsible for generating coercive attitudes towards bowel management in the parent. They are parental anxiety over the possible consequences of uncorrected chronic constipation; and parental insistence upon conformity of behaviour extending into the area of regular bowel acton.

Classically therefore, the personality profile to look out for is the rigid, perfectionist, pressurising parent, obsessionally clean and tidy, orderly to a fault, and insistent upon equivalent standards of personal hygiene in her children (Pinkerton, 1974).

Add to this domineering attitude an increasing sense of exasperation at the child's refusal to conform, and a vicious spiral is set up of increasingly hostile and coercive management meeting with increasingly stubborn resistance on the part of the toddler. Let no one underestimate either the chronicity or intractability of the problem engendered by this particular situation.

Persistence Beyond the Pre-School Stage

Nor is this pattern of management exclusively confined to the toddler age group. Although the history often goes back to when bowel control was first being achieved and additional emphasis was therefore being laid on bowel training, it is by no means uncommon to encounter obstipation apparently presenting in the middle years of childhood, even as late as 10 or 11; yet conflict over bowel training remains incriminated as the original issue. Predictably at this late stage, treatment will be especially difficult and protracted. In general, the more long standing and entrenched the functional bowel problem, the more problematic the prognosis and refractory the therapeutic response.

Organic v Functional

Bodian et al (1949) first demonstrated, at Great Ormond Street, the distinction between neurogenic megacolon, i.e. Hirschsprung's disease and what they termed 'idiopathic megacolon' due, in their opinion, to chronic colonic inertia. The so-called 'idiopathic' variety, although it ran a chronic course, was benign in its pathology, and unlike Hirschsprung's, did not warrant surgical intervention.

Our own study of intractable constipation based at Alder Hey Children's Hospital (Pinkerton, 1958) took this distinction one stage further. It suggested that the colonic inertia was actually secondary to long-standing bowel negativism of the type just described. Idiopathic megacolon is in fact psychogenic megacolon, and although benign in surgical terms, it is both more common than Hirschsprung's and by no means so benign in psychotherapeutic terms.

Moreover, even where the primary diagnosis *is* organic, and surgical intervention has been called for as in Hirschsprung's disease or other anatomical anomalies, parent/child conflict over bowel retraining may still complicate the issue and interfere profoundly with restoring bowel action despite successful surgery. In such cases, 'contamination' by secondary negativism more often leads to soiling than holding back of faeces; but both may equally detract from a successful surgical result.

Therapeutic Action

Where the diagnosis can be traced to ingrained bowel negativism, protracted treatment is the rule rather than the exception. Initially, enemata may have to be administered to clear the loaded bowel before rehabilitation can have any reasonable chance of succeeding. In these circumstances, particular care must be exercised against offending the child's dignity by conveying any impression of physical assault against his will. Thereby his already existing conflict with authority may be further inflamed.

Softening agents such as dioctyl sodium sulphosuccinate can be very helpful as an interim measure, if the child will accept them without suspicion. It is as well to

211

remember, however, that almost certainly he will have been pressurised at some previous stage into taking purgatives which may even have been camouflaged in his food or drink, so that he is understandably suspicious of any new approach.

It is imperative to gain his trust in any programme of psychotherapeutic re-habilitation designed to resolve long standing parent/child conflict. To this end, direct exhortation will almost certainly fall on deaf ears. He has heard it all before. The more effective approach is an oblique one through the medium of projective play therapy which encourages him to ventilate his feelings through an alternative channel of expression and so discharge them harmlessly. This technique calls for the specialised skills of a children's play therapist but is well worth considering in the long standing case. A variety of play procedures can be adopted; what they have in common is the opportunity for the child to act out his aggression vicari-ously.

In trying to promote parental insight for a change in management there is similarly no short cut. Long standing attitudes cannot be changed either by instant pronouncements or didactic advice. Any attempt to do so by prescribing a pro-gramme based on medical authority, will simply lead to the build up of parental resistance. This is usually covert rather than overt; it almost always remains polite, but it is no less dogged for all that.

The greatest mistake in these intractable cases is to underestimate the degree of negativism involved and its resistance to treatment; and thereby be tempted to adopt heroic measures of confrontation. They are almost certainly doomed to failure.

There is really no substitute for patient and painstaking counsel in re-educating the parental approach. This is undoubtedly slow, time consuming, repetitious, and as such, demanding of monumental patience; but nevertheless essential if it is going to work. When successful, it can be supremely rewarding.

References

Bodian, M, Stephens, S D and Ward, B C H (1949) *Lancet, i,* 6
Pinkerton, P (1958) *Archives of Disease in Childhood, 33,* 371
Pinkerton, P (1974) *Childhood Disorder – A Psychosomatic Approach .* Crosby Lockwood Staples, London. Pages 64 and 113
Thomas, A, Chess, S and Birch, H G (1968) *Temperament and Behaviour Disorders in Children.* University of London Press, London
Winnicott, D W (1958) *Through Paediatrics to Psychoanalysis.* Tavistock Publications, London

Surgical Management of Childhood Constipation

J LARI

In a paediatric practice, whether medical or surgical, many constipated children are seen, but in few is the constipation due to Hirschsprung's disease, the majority of whom present in the neonatal period. Only a few with short agang- lionic segment escape the net and present later as constipated children. For every one of these, many more present with the so-called functional megacolon. This group go under many headings, some of which are shown in Table I. I feel per- haps the last two on the list are the most precise, for these children have a grossly distended rectum which is inert from prolonged over-stretching.

TABLE I. Synonyms

Chronic Constipation
Idiopathic megacolon
Functional megacolon
Psychogenic megacolon
Colonic inertia
Pseudo-Hirschsprung's disease
Rectal inertia
Megarectum

A good and thorough history, a careful examination and a well supervised management of these children avoids many unnecessary barium enema examina- tions and cuts down the numbers of rectal biopsies. Table II shows the important salient differences between Hirschsprung's disease and chronic constipation (megarectum). The onset is perhaps the most important part of the history and not always easy to elucidate. I feel it is important to persist in one's inquiry and go into the neonatal history and find out when meconium was first passed. For in Hirschsprung's disease, there is a delay in passage of meconium beyond the first 24 hours in 94 per cent of cases (Swenson, 1973). So often parents use the term

213

	Hirschsprung's Disease	Chronic constipation Megarectum
Onset	Neonatal	Much later
Constipation	+	+
Distension	+	−
Soiling	−	+
Distal rectum	Empty	Loaded

'always' and 'as long as I can remember' but when one goes over it with them it becomes obvious that the child was all right in the first one or two years of life. Sometimes there is a precipitating cause like an illness or loss of someone dear to them. The basic problem appears to be persistent failure to respond to or resist the call to stool. An obvious example of resistance of call to stool is the child with fissure in ano, who resists the act of defaecation because of pain. Others for psychological reasons fail to respond to the call for defaecation.

Soiling or faecal incontinence is a common feature and sometimes the presenting symptom of megarectum, but it is usually absent in Hirschsprung's disease.

Distension is often gross in Hirschsprung's disease but absent in chronic constipation and, on rectal examination in the latter, one reaches the faecal mass straight away within 1 to 2 cm of anal verge; whereas in short segment Hirschsprung's disease, the 'anal canal' appears lengthened or the lower rectum is empty. This can sometimes be demonstrated by the radiologist with experience in this field by means of barium enema.

In cases where Hirschsprung's disease is suspected, these often include cases where the early history is missing, then a rectal biopsy differentiates the two conditions.

The diagnosis of Hirschsprung's disease rests ultimately on demonstrating the absence of ganglion cells. At most centres a full thickness rectal biopsy is required by the pathologist. This means the child needs a formal operation with general anaesthetics. It has been shown (Campbell & Noblett, 1969), that this is quite unnecessary and a simple suction biopsy of rectum will give a satisfactory answer in the majority of cases. This type of biopsy causes no more discomfort than a rectal examination and can be done as an outpatient procedure. Campbell and Noblett (1969) reported a successful diagnosis in 71 out of 85 patients, where an adequate biopsy was obtained. Certainly it is not difficult to recognise the normal where ganglion cells are in abundance. In Hirschsprung's disease many more serial sections from the specimen are required before a diagnosis of aganglionosis is reached. In difficult cases a formal full thickness biopsy could always be done.

214

Interpretation of rectal biopsy can be very difficult and is not always either black or white — there are grey areas. It is particularly in the interpretation of these grey areas that an experienced pathologist is most helpful, for it is not rare to find a child behaving like Hirschsprung's disease and yet ganglion cells are present. These may be few in number (hypoganglionosis); or vacuolated (degenerate cells); or the cells may be small and are called immature. I have seen several neonates with typical Hirschsprung's disease who required a colostomy, and a rectal biopsy showed immature ganglion cells. In the hope that with increased age the cells may have matured, the biopsies were repeated 6 to 12 months later, but these either showed no change or the picture became that of true aganglionosis.

The management of children with 'functional' constipation requires patience and careful explanation to the parents. I tell them that the child's rectal muscle has become over-stretched for so long that it has lost its tone and it will take time for it to come back to normal. Depending upon the severity, the child may require daily enemas at first, until the rectum is empty, then less frequent enemas, graduating to suppositories and aperients to ensure that the rectum is kept empty and gradually the muscle regains its tone. Depending on the severity and the conditions at home, some of these can be managed as outpatients but many require in-patient treatment.

The children with ultra-short segment Hirschsprung's disease are difficult to manage and may require formal resection of the aganglionosis segment. Some improve temporarily on anal dilatation. This has been noted in patients who had their anuses stretched incidently at the time of the rectal biopsy. A more permanent improvement occurs in some by excisional anorectal myotomy (Bentley, 1966). In this operation a longitudinal strip of internal anal sphincter and distal rectum is excised and the defect is sutured. In Bentley's series 10 out of 15 did well. Five had formal resection. Others like Duhamel (1966) have reported a similar degree of success.

In conclusion, the majority of children with constipation can be successfully treated by sympathetic but firm management. Very few require special investigation and a small number of these may need operative treatment.

References

Bentley, J F R (1966) *Archives of Disease of Childhood, 41,* 144
Campbell, P E, Noblett, H R (1969) *Journal of Paediatric Surgery, 4,* 410
Duhamel, B (1966) *Archives of Disease of Childhood, 41,* 150
Swenson, O, Sherman, J O, Fisher, J H (1973) *Journal of Paediatric Surgery, 8,* 587

Gastrointestinal Malignancies in Children

E N THOMPSON

Tumours in the gastrointestinal tract are relatively common in adults accounting for 30 to 40% of all fatal cancers in individuals over 30 years of age. In contrast, in children, only 1% of all malignancies develop at this site. Peller (1960) in a statistical analysis of all fatal malignant deaths in the US white population over a 5-year period, showed that 3.3% of childhood cancer deaths involved the gastrointestinal tract (including the mouth and pharynx) compared to 39.3% of all other age groups with a fatal cancer at this site. The rarity of cancer at this site in childhood is emphasised by the fact that from the entire tumour registry of more than 30,000 patients at the Yale—New Haven Hospital, only two patients were less than 16 years of age, one with a colonic cancer and the other a carcinoid tumour, found at appendectomy for acute appendicitis (Pickett & Briggs, 1967). Because of the extreme rarity of these cancers, they tend to be diagnosed late and generally carry a much worse prognosis than in adult patients. In addition to discussing cancers at different sites in the gastrointestinal tract, I intend to include other pathological conditions which are associated with a high cancer risk although this complication generally occurs in adult life.

OESOPHAGUS AND STOMACH

Primary oesphageal malignancy is extremely rare and in a world review by Moore only one definite case of squamous cell carcinoma and none of adenocarcinoma were found. In contrast the stomach is more commonly involved although in a total review of the world literature of 501 young people with gastric cancers only 19 were less than 15 years of age (McNeer, 1941). The presenting symptoms were pain, vomiting and weight loss, three-fourths of the patients had a palpable abdominal mass at presentation. The prognosis was appalling with a 6% 3 year survival rate.

216

SMALL INTESTINES

The commonest malignancy at this site is lymphosarcoma. Although an isolated primary lymphosarcoma may occur (ileal commoner than jejunal) the gastro-intestinal lesion is often part of a more generalised systemic disease, if not initially becoming so subsequently (Mestal, 1959). The treatment and prognosis is deter-mined by the presence or absence of co-existing generalised disease. These tumours can produce malabsorption, the mechanism thought to be due to infiltration of lymphatics with tumour.

Carcinoid tumours are found almost exclusively in the appendix in patients less than 20 years of age (Barclay & Robb, 1968) and are generally found at the time of appendectomy. In childhood these tumours are generally benign and localised. They are non-serotonin secreting and so do not give rise to the adult syndrome of patchy cyanosis, tachycardia, pulmonary stenosis, hyperperistalsis and diarrhoea. Polyposis of the small bowel is generally part of the Peutz Jeghers syndrome, a familial disorder characterised by buccal and circumoral pigmenta-tion, and hamartomatous polyps in the small intestine and stomach which may also occur in the large bowel. The polyps are not generally associated with any malignant change.

MALIGNANCY ASSOCIATED WITH CHRONIC SMALL BOWEL DISEASE

Coeliac Disease

For a long time the association between malabsorption and intestinal lymphomas has been known. However, in 1962 Gough and his colleagues reported the associa-tion of intestinal lymphoma and long standing coeliac disease and suggested an aetiological relationship. Since then other workers have confirmed the significantly increased incidence of lymphoma and adenocarcinoma within and outside the gastrointestinal tract (Harris et al, 1967; Kenwright, 1972; Barry & Read, 1973) in patients with long standing coeliac disease. Strict dietary control appeared to cor-relate with the incidence of neoplastic change (Harris et al, 1967). Asquith (1974) in a study of 208 patients found that it was possible to reduce the carcinoma but not lymphoma risk in those who had been treated with a strict gluten free diet for a minimum of 12 months. Whether long term treatment with gluten free diet will also reduce significantly the lymphoma risk is not yet known. However, in view of the known malignant association and the apparent greater risk in poorly controlled patients, it would seem wise to recommend strict dietary control in all patients with coeliac disease for life, until long term carefully controlled follow-up data is available. The mechanism for the malignant change is not known but such factors as defective epithelial cell maturation (Creamer, 1962), epithelial cell turnover (Croft et al, 1968), effects of chronic inflammation and, possibly, in-creased absorption of carcinogens from damaged mucosa (Kenrick & Walker-Smith,

1970) have been suggested. More recently it has been postulated that the defect in cell mediated and humerol immunity known to occur in these patients, is important in the development of neoplastic change (Maclaurin et al, 1971: Asquith, 1974).

Crohn's Disease

Malignant change in association with Crohn's disease has also been reported (Wyatt, 1969). As with coeliac disease the onset of the neoplasia occurred many years after the diagnosis of Crohn's disease. Adenocarcinoma and reticulum cell sarcoma were the malignant conditions noted. The mean duration of the symptoms of Crohn's disease was 15.7 years, and mean age of onset of neoplasia 42.7 years.

Colonic Lesions

In considering lesions at this site the question of polyposis has to be considered. Three types of polyps occur in paediatric patients, (1) juvenile polyps, (2) Peutz-Jeghers syndrome and (3) familial polyposis. Juvenile polyps are usually congenital hamartoma and occur principally in the rectum or colon. Similar polyps are found in the Peutz-Jeghers syndrome, although the polyps in this condition more commonly occur in the stomach and small bowel. Variable abdominal symptoms may be associated with both types of polyps but neoplastic change does not occur. Familial polyposis is inherited as a mendelian dominant trait, and affected individuals are at great risk from developing multi-focal carcinomatous changes within the polyps. The mean age of onset of symptoms of polyposis is 35 years of age (youngest reported with polyps and carcinoma 3 years). The mean age of onset of cancer is 42.9 years and death from this complication 43.9 years. Radical surgical therapy (proctocolectomy with ileostomy) has been recommended because of the very high cancer risk and appalling prognosis once established. Usually the children are diagnosed because an adult relative is found to have this disease. Because of the dominant mode of inheritance, careful screening of all members of the family is vital, remembering that the absence of polyps in young children does not exclude this diagnosis and continued serial examinations are necessary. In addition to the colonic neoplastic lesions, is the association of benign mesenchymal fibromas or lipomas in soft tissue and bone as in Gardner's syndrome, malignant mesenchymal tumours (Fraumeni et al, 1968) and brain tumours (Turcott et al, 1959). Another disorder associated with a high risk of colonic cancer is ulcerative colitis (Edwards & Truelove, 1964; Goligher et al, 1968; Devroede et al, 1971). Devroede et al (1971) in a study of 396 children with ulcerative colitis followed up for 6 to 43 years, noted a cancer risk of 20% per decade after the first decade, although 3% developed cancer during the first 10 years of the disease. The age of onset of colitis did not affect overall survival but patients aged between 5 and 9 years had the highest cancer risk. Patients with widespread colonic involvement had a higher risk than those with localised rectal involvement, but these patients were more at risk than normal individuals, with a risk similar to that in patients with familial polyposis. They predicted that only 50% of those with rectal involvement would be alive 40 years after onset of the colitis, emphasising the need to take the cancer risk seriously. They noted no change in the cancer risk pattern since the steroid era, although this therapy had affected the initial colitis mortality. In another large British study (Edwards & Truelove, 1964) the following poor prognostic factors were noted; age of onset, continuous disease, widespread involvement and clinical severity of the first attack. They felt that if one or more of these factors, *especially* onset in childhood were present, early radical surgery should be seriously considered (i.e. within 10 years of the onset of symptoms). Thus both these groups have stressed the need for early surgery (proctocolectomy with ileostomy) despite the well known high mortality in the first post-operative year, because after the first year the predicted life expectancy is no different from normal children (Daly, 1968; Devroede et al, 1971).

Carcinoma of the colon and rectum can occur independently of familial polyposis and ulcerative colitis; 200 such patients reported in the world literature were reviewed by O'Brien (1967). The age distribution ranged from infancy upwards, but 80% were 10 to 16 years old. The majority of cancers were in the rectum. Half of the tumours were mucoid adenocarcinomas, which is interesting when compared with an incidence of 5% in adults. The outlook of these children was bad, possibly due to delay in diagnosis and widespread involvement at the time of presentation.

THE LIVER

This is an uncommon site for tumours in infants and children but frequent enough to be considered as a major diagnostic problem in children with an abdominal mass. These lesions may be benign or malignant; the former hamartomas, the latter hepatoblastomas, hepatocellular carcinomas or rhabdomyosarcomas. The age of onset of hepatomas is related to histological classification. Hepatoblastomas and benign hamartoma are almost always found in infants less than 2 years whereas hepatocellular carcinomas generally occur in children over 5 years (Keeling, 1970). Hepatomas are much less frequent than other embryonal tumours except in the newborn period when they are found more frequently than at any other time in childhood (Fraumeni et al, 1968). Treatment of primary hepatomas is surgical although the outlook is poor (Raffuci & Ramirez-Schon, 1970) despite a tendency to late metastases. Aggressive surgery is possible because of the tremendous capacity of the child's liver to regenerate. Cancer chemotherapy and irradiation do not play a role in therapy. However, there have been encouraging recent reports of the value of adriamycin in hepatocellular carcinoma.

219

SUMMARY

Cancer of the gastrointestinal tract is a rarity in childhood. Colonic lesions occur most frequently, with the exception of lymphosarcoma in the small intestine, which may be primary or part of a more generalised systemic process. Adenomatous polyps, particularly multiple or familial, should be regarded as potentially malignant. The potential malignant change in coeliac disease, Crohn's disease and ulcerative colitis should be appreciated and the importance of dietary control in the former and radical surgery within 10 years of the onset of colitis seriously considered in the management of such patients. The prognosis of established gastrointestinal cancer in childhood is very poor and much worse than adult cancer at similar sites.

References

Asquith, P (1974) *Proceedings of the 2nd International Coeliac Symposium.* (Ed) W Th, Hekkens, J M Peña, A S Stenfert Kroese. Page 321

Asquith, P (1974) Ibid. Page 246

Barclay, G P T, Robb, W A T (1968) *Surgery, Gynecology and Obstetrics, 126,* 483

Barry, R E and Read, A E (1973) *Quarterly Journal of Medicine, 42,* 665

Creamer, B (1962) *Gut, 3,* 295

Croft, D N, Loehry, C A and Creamer, B (1968) *Lancet, ii,* 68

Daly, D W (1968) *Annals of the Royal College of Surgeons of England, 42,* 38

Devroede, G H, Taylor, W F, Sauerw, G, Jackman, R J and Stickler, G B (1971) *285,* 17

Edwards, F C and Truelove, S C, (1964) *Gut, 5,* 15

Fraumeni, J F J, Vogel, ChL and Easton, J M (1968) *Archives of Internal Medicine, 121,* 57

Fraumeni, J F, Miller, R W and Hill, J F (1968) *Journal of the National Cancer Institute, 40,* 1087

Gardner, E J and Richards, R C (1953) *American Journal of Human Genetics, 5,* 139

Goligher, J C, de Dombal, F T, Watts, J Mck et al (1968) *Ulcerative Colitis,* Baillière Tindal and Cassell, London

Gough, K R, Read, A E and Naish, J M (1962) *Gut, 3,* 232

Harris, O D, Cooke, W T, Thompson, H and Waterhouse, R (1967) *American Journal of Medicine, 42,* 899

Keeling, J (1970) *Journal of Pathology, 103,* 69

Kenrick, K G and Walker-Smith, J A (1970) *Gut, 11,* 635

Kenwright, S (1972) *Postgraduate Medical Journal, 48,* 673

Maclaurin, B P, Cooke, W T and Ling, N R (1971) *Gut, 12,* 794

McNeer, G (1941) *American Journal of Roentgenology, 45,* 537

Mestal, A L (1959) *American Surgeon, 149,* 87

Moore, C (1958) *Paediatrics, 21,* 573

O'Brien, S E (1967) *Canadian Medical Association Journal, 96,* 1217

Peller, S (1960) *Cancer in Childhood and Youth.* John Wright & Sons Ltd, Bristol

Pickett, L K and Briggs, H C (1967) *Pediatric Clinics of North America, 14,* 223

Raffuci, F L and Ramirez-Schon, G (1970) *Surgery, Gynecology and Obstetrics, 130,* 371

Turcot, J., Despres, J P, St. Pierre, F (1959) *Disease of the Colon and Rectum, 2,* 465

Wyatt, A P (1969) *Gut, 10,* 924

Discussion

MR FREEMAN Is there any evidence to show whether meticulous attention to a gluten free diet reduces the risk of carcinoma?

PROFESSOR HADORN There was a recent symposium on coeliac disease, and a paper was presented which showed that the incidence of lymphoma did not appear to be influenced by the dietary treatment, whereas incidence of other cancers seemed to be much lower in patients who were maintained on a strict gluten-free diet.

DR NELSON I was wondering whether the answer to this will come in the next decade. In adult coeliac disease, it appears that treatment does not influence the cancer risk, whereas we are only in the future going to see the effects of treating childhood coeliac disease from early infancy. I suppose we will now be coming up to the time when sufficient patients will be available to answer these questions.

DR DODGE I think this is a very important point because the recent study by McCrae and colleagues in Edinburgh (1975) showed that the vast majority of patients who have spontaneously come off a gluten-free diet were in perfectly good health many years later.

References

McCrae, W M, Eastwood, M A, Martin, M R and Sircus, W (1975) *Lancet, i,* 187

Panel Discussion
CONSTIPATION

MR LARI   Could you discuss the concept of ultra-short segment Hirschsprung's disease? It is a practical problem because one of the things that influence you in further investigation is what you feel when you put your finger in the rectum.

MR FREEMAN   Before I ask Mr Howard to answer that I would like to comment that differences between Hirschsprung's disease and chronic constipation are no longer as clear as you implied. Sometimes children with Hirschsprung's disease do soil, and in some you can feel faeces right down at the recto-anal margin. I am not sure that you can always get enough clinical information. From what Mr Howard said, the 'grey area' around the internal sphincter 2-4 cm above the internal sphincter is not normally innervated with the ganglion cells you see above, and I think with due respect you cannot diagnose the ultra-short segments involving internal sphincter only by biopsy.

MR HOWARD   I think that is a very fair comment. I feel sceptical of short-segment Hirschsprung's disease as described, and I think this is one of the areas where you need to know your pathologist well. If a pathologist just looks at these things occasionally, it is very difficult for him to get a concept of what the range is in the lower part of the rectum as far as normal histology goes. There is remarkably little work actually done on this, the biggest difficulty is getting normal material.

LARI   Mr Chairman, I think this question of ultra-short segment Hirschsprung's disease is confused because some people's ultra-short is not other people's ultra-short. Yours is just the anal canal, others is perhaps the lower rectum as well. I agree that some of the cases are very difficult, and if one has grounds to do manometry then that is fine. I find usually that when a child has to undergo manometry it is very difficult, you first have to let him get used to your instruments.

222

HOWARD   Yes, you must have time, you cannot just rush into it.

DR BURMAN   If you cannot diagnose this condition histologically, why do you call it Hirschsprung's disease and not describe it in manometric terms?

FREEMAN   I think that is fair comment. Perhaps you can call it achalasia as some people have suggested. Whatever you name it, there is a non-relaxing internal sphincter which has the symptomatology of Hirschsprung's disease.

BURMAN   It produces constipation and biometric changes. Surely Hirschsprung's disease means a histological abnormality, which is not demonstrable in these so-called ultra-short segments? Therefore could not this be a functional condition, with perhaps psychiatric origin, because all you are showing is a manometric change, not a histological change?

FREEMAN   Perhaps I should not answer that, but it is relieved by extended sphincterotomy. If you incise the internal sphincter you will cure the condition in the majority of cases. In Hirschsprung's disease sometimes a Swenson operation removes it to within about a centimetre of the anus, and leaves a ganglionic bowel which is no different from the ultra-short segment. Now a lot of these cases did not benefit until you went back and divided half the internal sphincter or stretched it. There is therefore a pathological area at this site. I think also that punch biopsies are often inadequate for most pathologists, because you are uncertain about the exact level from which they have been obtained and if ganglion cells are about it may be difficult to interpret.

PROFESSOR HADORN   I think that in small biopsies you are unlikely to miss the enormous increase in fibres if you do the cholinesterase stain. Our surgeons say that if they do this systematically by the method of Meier-Ruge in Basle they are very satisfied and we do not do full thickness surgical biopsies any more.

FREEMAN   I think the vast majority of cases which we are talking about can be sorted out fairly easily. But there is a hard core of intractable constipation where you need not only the Special Centres but the superspecialists who are prepared to do the manometry and the cholinesterase stains and all the other stains, otherwise you are not going to get your answers.
   Does anybody know what happens to the chronic constipations when they grow up? Either the paediatricians treat them very effectively or else something else happens, but we do not seem to see them in adult life.

HOWARD   I followed up a group of Mr Nixon's patients and of about 15 of them 14 seem to be normal now. I cannot explain this, I cannot even say at what age they started to co-operate or what happens. Adult constipation seems to come on later, doesn't it?

DR DODGE I think it is important to know this natural history because we can reassure the parents of children with encopresis and dilated rectums that they will eventually grow out of it. It is said that they all grow out of it by the age of 14, although this is not very much encouragement for the parents of encopretic 6-year olds.

DR PINKERTON Although I would in general agree with that, there were in our original series three children who went on to the age of 16 or more with constipation and eventually had to have hemicolectomies. Only this week I saw another 16-year old who we first picked up when she was five. The psychopathology there is intractable, but in general, rather like the asthmatics, they do seem to lose their symptoms both physiologically and psycho-physiologically.

FREEMAN There was a paper from St Mark's where they found that 20% of adult megacolons turned out to have Hirschsprung's disease.

COMMENT FROM AUDIENCE They see things at St Mark's which other gastroenterologists do not see anywhere else.

FREEMAN We often talk rather glibly about anal fissures producing constipation in children, but which is the chicken and which is the egg? I mean why do they get anal fissures, and why do they start on the cycle?

DR PROSSER You also see fissures in patients who do not have constipation or pain.

FREEMAN There is considerable disagreement. Some people say that they always have pain, others say they don't.

DR LEWIS I would like to ask Dr Howard how long it takes for cathartic colon to develop. Is there any way of getting round this in patients by the intermittent use of Senokot?

HOWARD It seems to take about 10 years. I do use Senokot; I think it is a very useful drug, but it should be given in short courses. You would be surprised how long some of the patients attending St Mark's have been on cathartics. Perhaps we should switch the discussion a little on to what should be the management of these children. We have heard about the dangers of enemas and suppositories, but what should we be doing?

PINKERTON As Mr Lari has said, whatever may be the psychological factors involved, attention to this aspect will not unbind a bound up colon. It is im-

224

portant to remember that management is not only conducted in Super Centres but also in the periphery and that there may be badly managed enemata or laxatives or suppositories and that when a child shrinks from you it may be because you are the last person in a long line to have greeted him. You would be amazed at some of the stories they may have been told before they get to you. We have found an emulsifying agent like dioctyl sodium succinate very helpful in keeping the faeces soft, rather than something more active like Senokot. I think if you talk to the child and his parents and try to clarify the situation, you will find they are more co-operative. I think it is the approach rather than what you do which is important. I think that by these means you can get even the most recalcitrant child to take what was obnoxious to him before. I accept that in these chronic cases you have to work with physical means before you can get started on psychotherapeutic rehabilitation.

FREEMAN We have neglected something which was mentioned, namely the business of the toilet, and the flushing and the frightening experience, and I think that this is where a lot of childhood constipation starts. In Africa where it is warm and dry, the child defaecates behind a bush and takes a diet with plenty of fibre, and there is no problem of chronic constipation. I think the social conditions are an area we must pay more attention to. If the child lives in a house with only an outside toilet and it is cold in Winter, or goes to school where there are no doors on the toilets, then he will not defaecate. I think that a massive campaign on the school toilets in this country would take away probably 70% of the chronic constipation problems.

DR HARRIES I wonder whether any of the adult gastroenterologists here have encountered problems of laxative-induced chronic diarrhoea in adults which started in childhood?

DR MORRIS We have certainly encountered adult patients with chronic diarrhoea who are suspected of having an endocrine tumour and when you look in their lockers you find the reason for their diarrhoea, because they are full of laxatives.

LEWIS I would like to ask whether anyone has ever tried an artificial diet in the initial treatment of these patients with a decompression of the large bowel?

DODGE One of the problems with treating these children with an artificial diet is that it might be seen as a punishment as it is so unpleasant but there are more palatable preparations coming on the market, and I think that this is quite a useful suggestion.

BURMAN This is suggesting that the basic problem is contracting of the bowel, but I thought most people would agree that this is not the case.

225

HOWARD The suggestion is that you use it in the initial phase and that it is an aid to helping the bowel contract. We have actually used it in one or two cases just on common sense principles to try to reduce the residue, and it worked well.

DR NELSON Our experience in the North East where chronic constipation seems to be very common is that it is essentially a psychological problem. Psychotherapy very often seems to produce a substitution of symptoms and I was impressed by the number of children who get into trouble with authority, even though we have cured their constipation. Have you experienced this in Liverpool?

PINKERTON Yes, I think we have observed the same thing, that we are simply substituting one sympton for another. Unless you resolve the conflict you are going to get other problems and this is exactly what I think would happen with your artificial diet.

DR LITTLEWOOD I would just like to take up this point about the young babies who have a bowel very different from that of other babies in that they are constipated. In spite of the emphasis which has been placed on the psychological side, which I agree is very important, I think that there is basically an organic problem which can be conditioned into appearance by negativism.

PINKERTON That is a very interesting idea, and I agree that there is a group of babies who have constipation or sluggish bowels which is constitutional. It is often familial and comes down again to management because if you do not make an issue of it, it can be quite reasonably controlled. In our original study we found that those who went on to develop megacolon or megarectum were those where the matter had been made an issue by the parents or by the physician or both. If we left them alone and made no issue of it there was no recurrence. I am not going into the details of the pathophysiology, I think if you let nature takes its course it will right itself.